Bread Cookbook 2021

Delicious Baking Recipes with Step-by-Step Tutorials on How to Make any Loaf of Bread

Table of Contents

INTRODUCTION 4

CRANBERRY ORANGE QUICK BREAD 6

CHOCOLATE CHIP AND PUMPKIN BREAD 8

SUPER MOIST PUMPKIN BREAD 10

APPLESAUCE PUMPKIN SPICE BREAD 12

TOASTED PECAN BUTTER 14

PUMPKIN-CREAM CHEESE MINI LOAVES 16

CHOCOLATE ZUCCHINI BREAD 18

LEMON PISTACHIO ZUCCHINI BREAD 20

BLUEBERRY ZUCCHINI BREAD 22

ZUCCHINI BREAD WITH COCONUT 24

PINEAPPLE COCONUT ZUCCHINI BREAD 26

BANANA-ZUCCHINI BREAD 28

ZUCCHINI APPLE BREAD 30

HARVEST VEGETABLE BREAD 32

HEARTY BREAKFAST MUFFINS 34

SAVORY CHEDDAR ZUCCHINI MUFFINS 36

KINGMAN'S VEGAN ZUCCHINI BREAD 38

JALAPENO GREEN ONION ALE CORN BREAD 40

SWEET CORN CAKE 42

HONEY CORNBREAD 44

BLUEBERRY CORNBREAD 46

ABSOLUTE MEXICAN CORNBREAD 48

EXCELLENT AND HEALTHY CORNBREAD 50

GOLDEN SWEET CORNBREAD 52

VEGAN JALAPENO CORNBREAD IN THE AIR FRYER 54

ANGIE'S DILLY CASSEROLE BREAD 56

ZA'ATAR PULL-APART BREAD ROLLS 58

LEBANESE MOUNTAIN BREAD 60

MUSTARD WHEAT RYE SANDWICH BREAD 62

MONKEY BREAD 64

WHOLE WHEAT HONEY BREAD 66

LIGHT WHEAT BREAD ROLLS 68

FLAX AND SUNFLOWER SEED BREAD 70

DEE'S HEALTH BREAD 72

SEVEN GRAIN BREAD 74

CRACKED WHEAT SOURDOUGH BREAD 76

WHOLE WHEAT SEED BREAD 78

SIMPLE WHOLE WHEAT BREAD 80

SAN FRANCISCO SOURDOUGH BREAD 82

PLAIN AND SIMPLE SOURDOUGH BREAD 84

FRENCH COUNTRY BREAD 86

NO-KNEAD ARTISAN STYLE BREAD 88

AUTHENTIC GERMAN BREAD (BAUERNBROT) 90

HONEY BUNCH BREAD 92

CHEF JOHN'S CUBAN BREAD 94

BLENDER WHITE BREAD 97

BUTTERMILK BREAD 99

TRADITIONAL WHITE BREAD 101

CIABATTA 103

ONION BREAD 106

INTRODUCTION

You've just stepped into a whole new world of pleasure and a nutritious diet that will help you satisfy both your taste buds and your health requirements. This book will provide you with delectable bread-making recipes, as well as a step-by-step tutorial on how to produce each form of bread and its nutritional value.

First, let's look at the health implications of a bread-based diet.

In the year 2020, about 200 million Americans consumed one package of bread each week on average. With so many homes relying on bread products for their daily meals, the nutritional worth of bread is called into doubt. If you or your family consumes bread on a daily basis, or even on rare occasions, you should be aware of its nutritional value. Explore this guide to learn about the health advantages of bread, as well as the bread nutrition of many goods you presumably consume on a daily basis.

Bread is a pantry essential for many people. They virtually always have it on available and use it in all of their meals. Whether you toast it, make sandwiches with it, or use it in a variety of dishes, you may wonder, "Is bread healthy?" Given the variety of bread kinds and types available, it's preferable not to respond with a blanket "yes." Varied types of bread, however, have different health benefits.

Overall, the goods you select decide whether or not bread is healthy. You want products that are manufactured with high-quality ingredients and come from a reputable company. The way you eat bread goods has an impact on your health as well. Bread, like anything else, should be consumed in moderation to avoid any negative consequences. Depending on what else you consume and the type of bread product you prefer, some experts recommend restricting yourself to one serving of bread each meal or per day. Check the nutrition facts on the bread and, depending on your diet, follow the serving instructions or eat less at a time.

This book is the greatest choice for you if you really want to avoid any health dangers while eating your beloved bread because it offers all of the healthy bread-making methods. If you follow the instructions in this book, the following are some of the advantages of eating bread!

Bread Contains Fiber

Bread Contains Protein

Bread Can Decrease the Risk of Cancer

Bread Can Be Enriched with Micronutrients

Bread Has a Prebiotic Effect

Bread Is Low in Fat

Bread Fuels Your Body

Now that you've learned about the health benefits of bread, it's time to learn how to make it so that you may reap all of the benefits. So, let's get to work.

CRANBERRY ORANGE QUICK BREAD

Preparation: 15 Minutes

Cook: 20 Minutes

Servings: 10

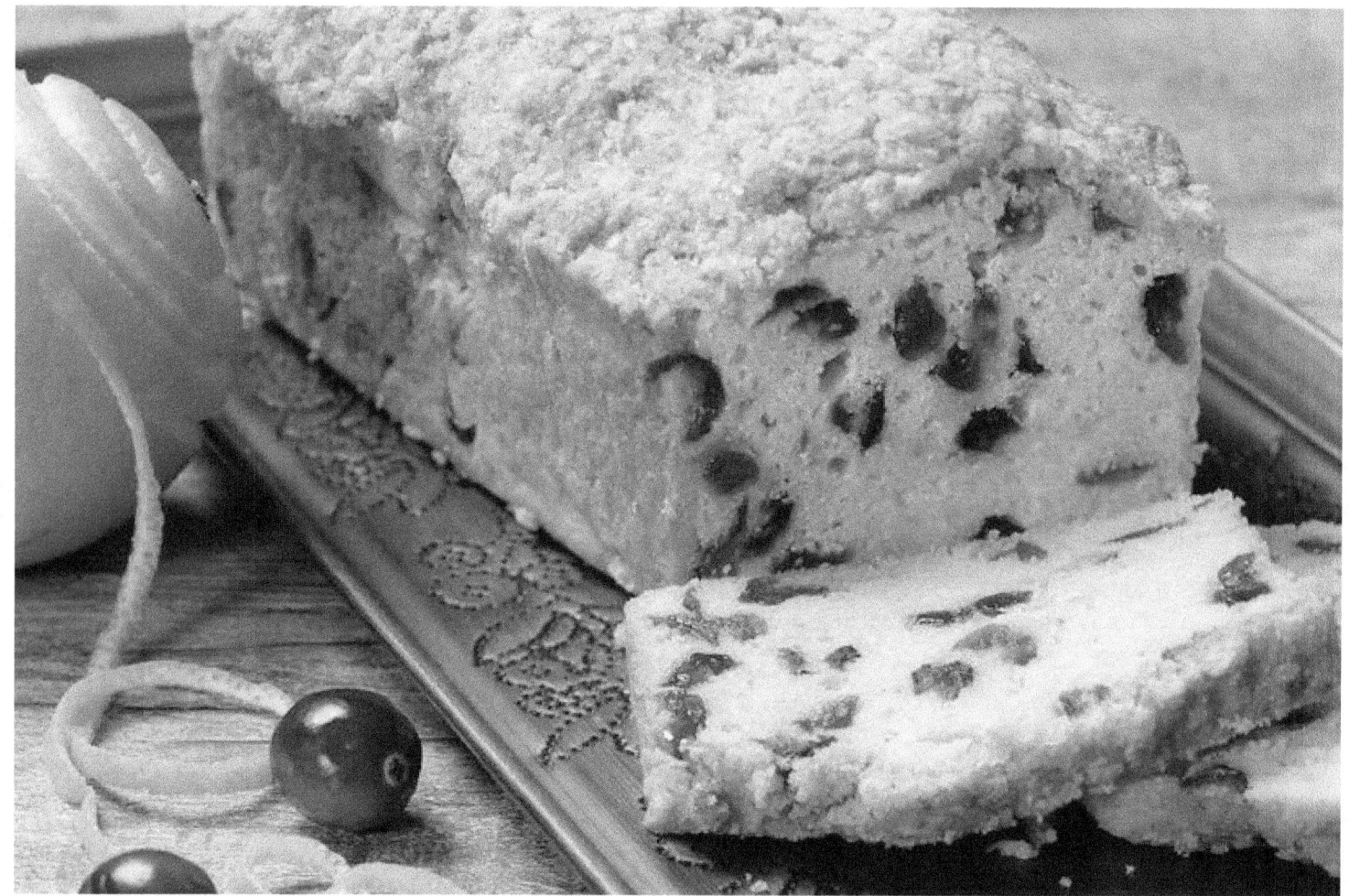

Breakfast, lunch, or just a snack, this rich and hearty fruit bread is perfect. For Thanksgiving, my in-laws devoured it.

Nutrition

Calories: 212 | Protein: 3.1g | Cholesterol: 35.3mg | Sodium: 159mg

Carbohydrates: 33.9g | Fat: 7.3g

Ingredients

- 2 eggs
- 2 cups cranberries
- ¾ cup milk
- 1 ¾ cups white sugar
- ¼ teaspoon baking soda
- ½ cup butter, melted
- 1 teaspoon vanilla extract
- 1 cup mandarin orange segments, drained
- 2 ¾ cups all-purpose flour
- 2 teaspoons baking powder
- 1 teaspoon orange extract
- ½ teaspoon salt
- ¾ cup sour cream

Instructions

1. Preheat the oven to 350°F. Grease two 8x4 inch loaf pans. Combine the flour, baking powder, baking soda, salt, and white sugar in a large mixing bowl. Add the melted butter and stir until the mixture is crumbly. Mix the cranberries and oranges in a mixing bowl. Whisk together the eggs, milk, sour cream, vanilla, and orange essence in a separate dish or large measuring cup.
2. . Pour the liquid components into the dry ingredients bowl and mix briefly to combine. Using a spatula, evenly distribute the batter across the prepared pans.
3. Bake for forty minutes in a preheated oven or until a toothpick inserted into the crown comes out clean. Allow it to cool in the pans for a few minutes before removing to wire racks to cool fully.

CHOCOLATE CHIP AND PUMPKIN BREAD

Preparation: 15 Minutes

Cook: 1 Hour

Servings: 20

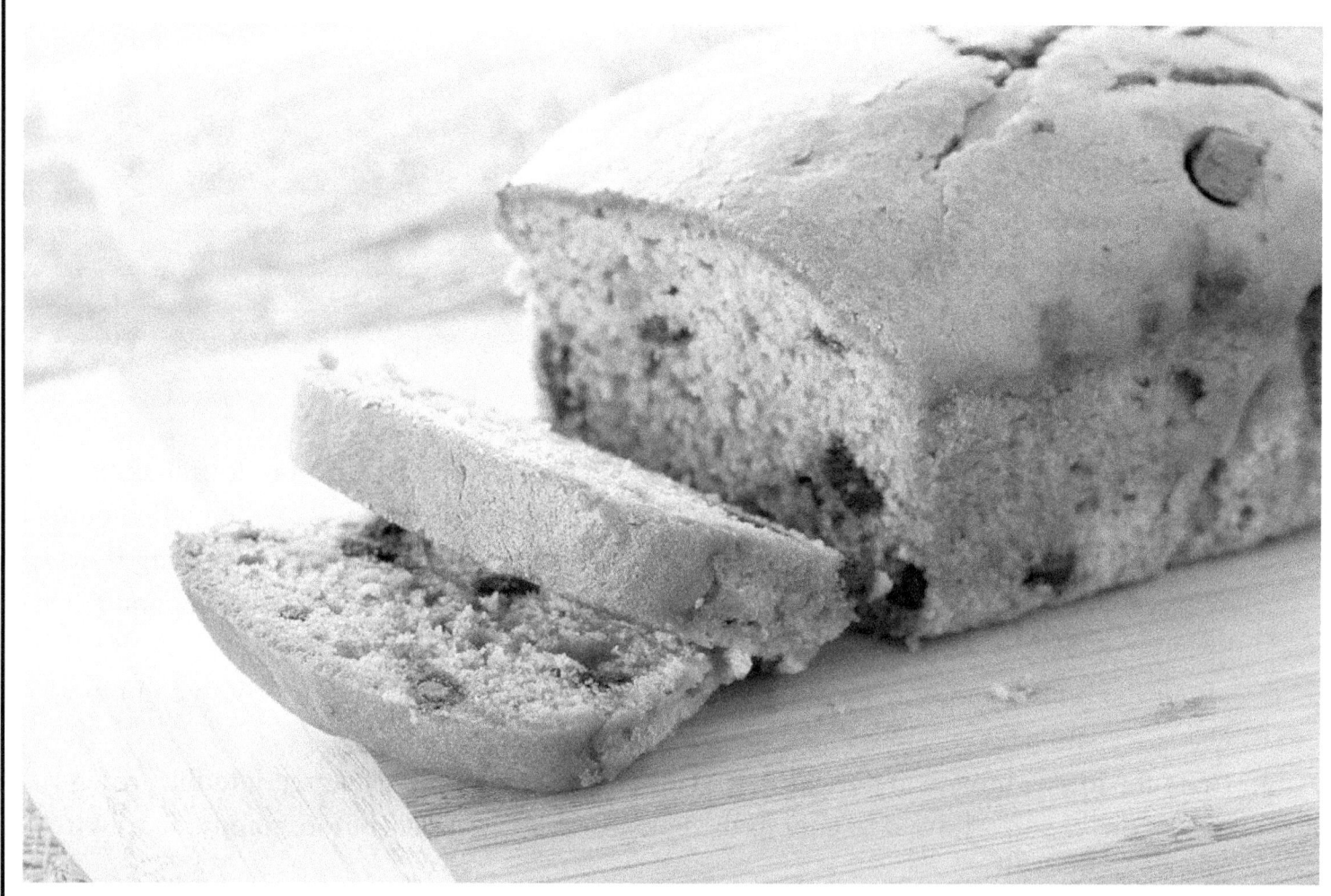

Pumpkin bread that is moist and delicious. Breakfast or dessert, this dish is delicious. A seasonal favorite or year-round delight. Kid-approved!

Nutrition

Calories: 343 | Protein: 4.3g | Cholesterol: 37.2mg | Sodium: 307.4mg

Carbohydrates: 50.9g | Fat: 15.3g

Ingredients

- 1 package semisweet chocolate chips
- cooking spray
- 4 eggs, beaten
- 3 cups self-rising flour
- ⅔ cup vegetable oil
- 1 can pumpkin puree
- 2 teaspoons vanilla extract
- 1 cup white sugar
- 1 cup brown sugar
- 2 teaspoons pumpkin pie spice

Instructions

1. Preheat the oven to 350 degrees Fahrenheit. Using cooking spray, coat two 9x5-inch loaf pans.
2. In a mixing bowl, combine the pumpkin puree, white sugar, brown sugar, eggs, vegetable oil, vanilla extract, and pumpkin pie spice; add the flour and mix until a dough form. Whisk in the chocolate chips and divide the batter between the two loaf pans.
3. Bake for one hour in a preheated oven or until a toothpick inserted in the center comes out clean. Before taking the bread from the pans, let it cool for fifteen minutes.

SUPER MOIST PUMPKIN BREAD

Preparation: 15 Minutes

Cook: 1 Hour

Servings: 20

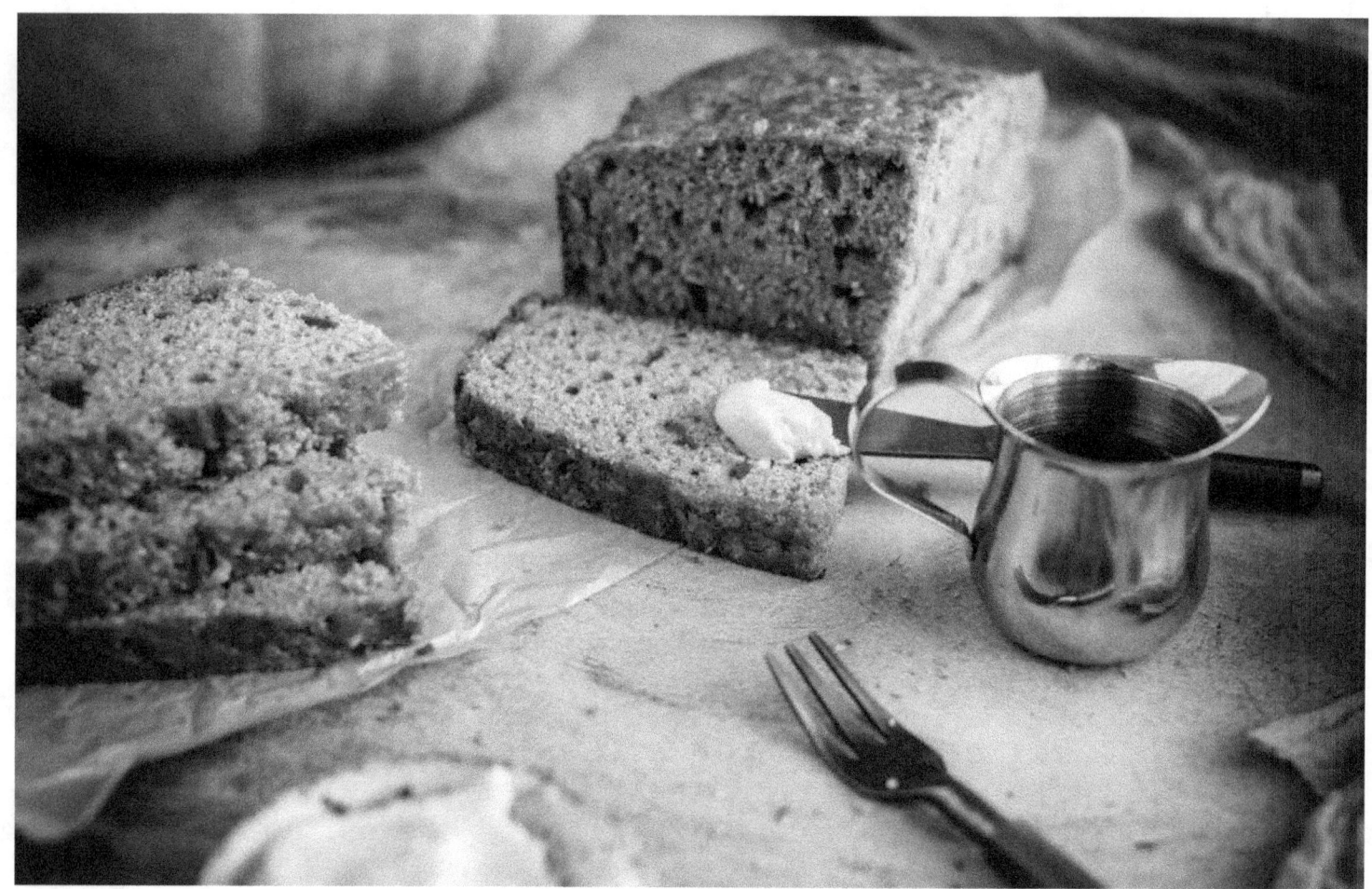

This is a fantastic loaf of bread. Its moistness is due to the use of a unique ingredient: milk made from coconut

Nutrition

Calories: 360 | Protein: 3.6g | Fat: 17.7g | Sodium: 257.4mg | Carbohydrates: 48.9g

Ingredients

- 3 ½ cups all-purpose flour
- 2 cups packed dark brown sugar
- ⅔ cup white sugar
- 2 cups pumpkin puree
- 1 cup vegetable oil
- ⅔ cup coconut milk
- 2 teaspoons baking soda
- 1 teaspoon salt
- 1 teaspoon ground nutmeg
- 1 ½ teaspoon ground cinnamon
- ⅔ cup flaked coconut
- 1 cup toasted walnuts, chopped

Instructions

1. Preheat the oven to 350 degrees Fahrenheit. Two 8x4 inch loaf pans should be greased and floured.
2. Mix the flour, brown sugar, white sugar, pumpkin puree, oil, coconut milk, baking soda, salt, ground nutmeg, and ground cinnamon together in a large mixing bowl. Mix until the flour is completely gone. Combine the nuts and flaked coconut in a mixing bowl. Pour the batter into the pans that have been prepared.
3. Bake for one hour and fifteen minutes at 350 degrees F, or until a toothpick inserted in the center comes out clean. Remove the loaves from the oven and wrap them tightly in foil. Allow ten minutes for steaming. Remove the foil and place the cake on a cooling rack. Allow it to cool entirely after lightly tenting with foil.

APPLESAUCE PUMPKIN SPICE BREAD

Preparation: 15 Minutes

Cook: 1 Hour

Servings: 24

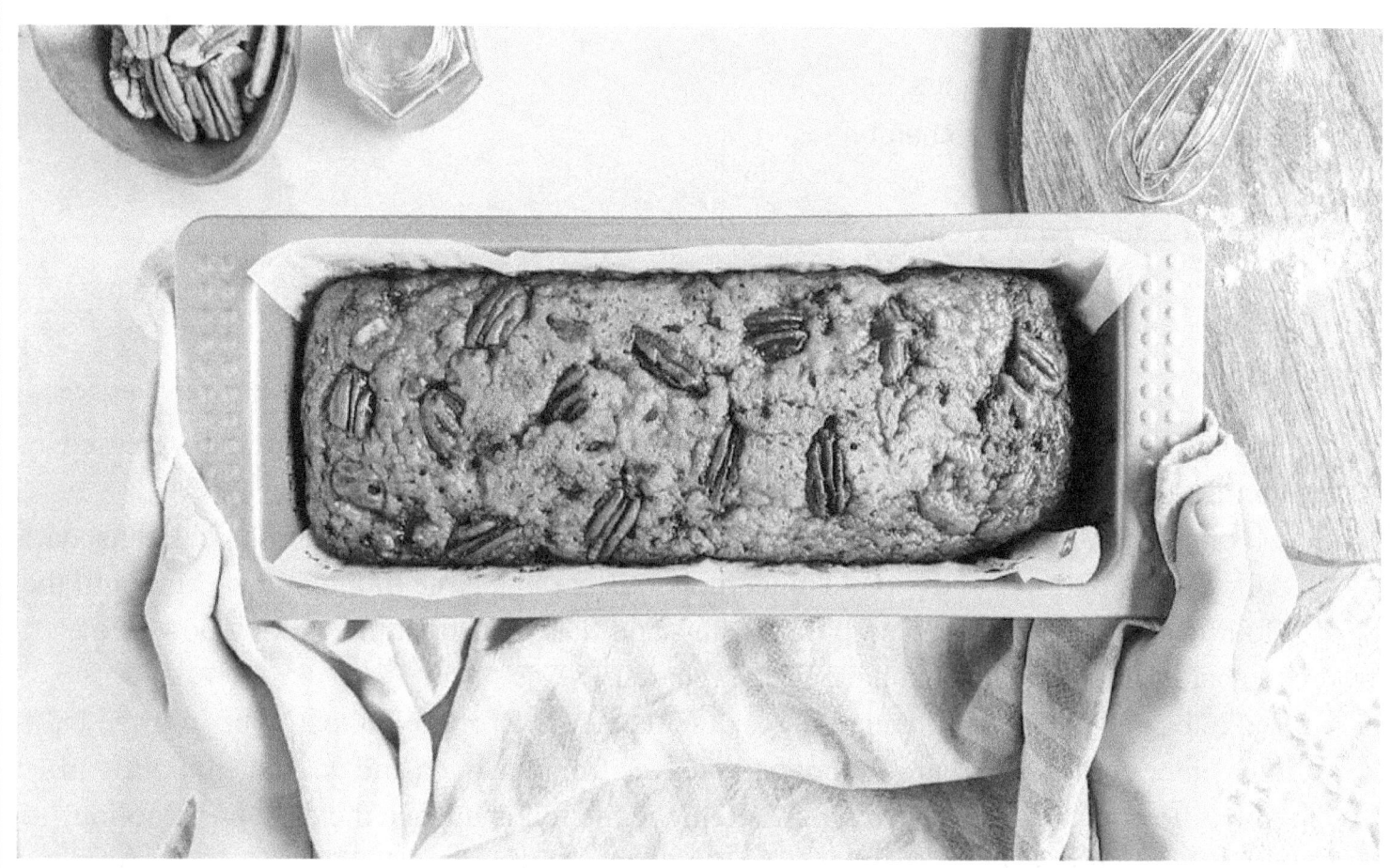

This is one of my favorite holiday dishes! It stays well and is an excellent dish to serve at holiday celebrations.

Nutrition

Calories: 197 | Protein: 3.3g | Cholesterol: 31mg | Sodium: 220.4mg

Carbohydrates: 44g | Fat: 1.3g

Ingredients

- 3 ½ cups unbleached all-purpose flour
- 4 eggs, lightly beaten
- 1 ½ tablespoon ground nutmeg
- cooking spray
- ½ cup water
- 1 teaspoon baking soda
- 1 cup unsweetened applesauce
- 1 teaspoon salt
- 2 cups dark brown sugar
- 1 cup white sugar
- 1 teaspoon ground ginger
- ½ teaspoon baking powder
- 3 tablespoons ground cinnamon
- 2 teaspoons ground cloves
- 1 can solid-pack pumpkin

Instructions

1. Preheat the oven to 350 degrees Fahrenheit. Take 2 loaf pans and sprayed them with cooking spray.
2. In a large mixing bowl, combine flour, cinnamon, nutmeg, cloves, ginger, baking soda, salt, and baking powder.
3. In a large mixing bowl, combine brown sugar, white sugar, applesauce, and eggs. Mix in the pumpkin thoroughly. Alternate adding the flour mixture and the water, mixing well after each addition. Divide the batter amongst the loaf pans that have been prepped.
4. Bake the loaves in the preheated oven for sixty to sixty-five minutes, or until a toothpick inserted in the center comes out clean. Allow ten minutes for cooling in the pans. To cool entirely, invert onto a wire rack.

TOASTED PECAN BUTTER

Preparation: 5 Minutes

Cook: 15 Minutes

Servings: 32

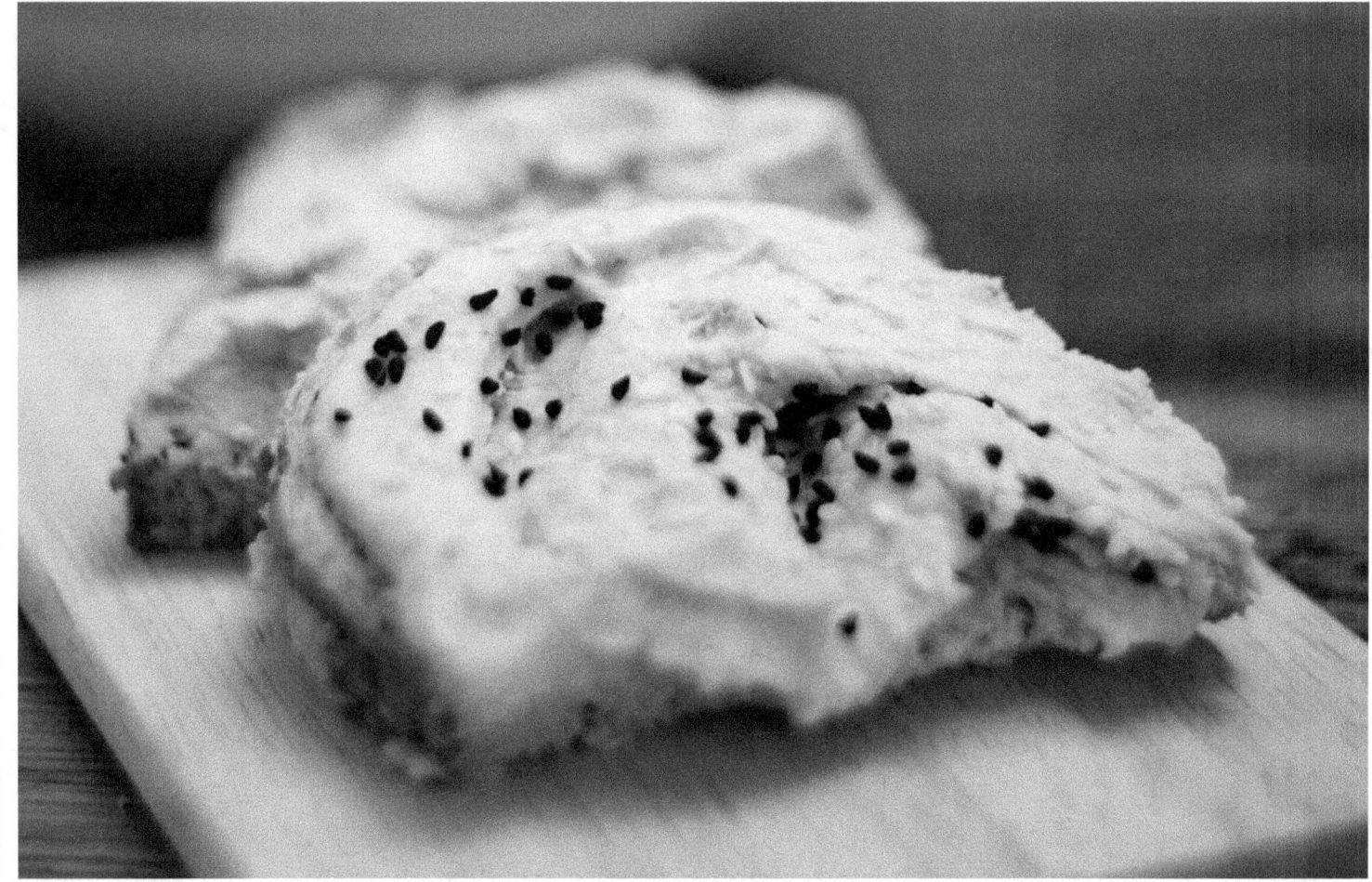

This is a fantastic addition to holiday brunches. Serve with bread, buns, and biscuits, if desired. On pancakes, waffles, and croissants, it's delicious!

Nutrition

Calories: 67 | Protein: 0.2g | Cholesterol: 15.3mg | Sodium: 41.2mg

Carbohydrates: 1.4g | Fat: 7g

Ingredients

- 1 cup butter at room temperature
- 1 teaspoon vanilla extract
- ¼ cup light brown sugar
- ½ cup chopped pecans

Instructions

1. Preheat the oven to 325 degrees Fahrenheit/165 degrees Celsius.
2. Spread the pecans out on a baking sheet and toast in a preheated oven for about fifteen minutes, or until golden brown and aromatic. As they bake, keep an eye on them since they burn quickly. Allow it to cool to room temperature before serving.
3. To completely incorporate the brown sugar, butter, and vanilla in a food processor, pulse several times. The butter will have a slight fluffiness to it. Toss in the cooled nuts and pulse a few times to incorporate. Pulse the pecans a few more times for a finer grind. Serve right away, or store in a jar with a lid in the refrigerator.

PUMPKIN-CREAM CHEESE MINI LOAVES

Preparation: 20 Minutes

Cook: 25 Minutes

Total: 55 Minutes

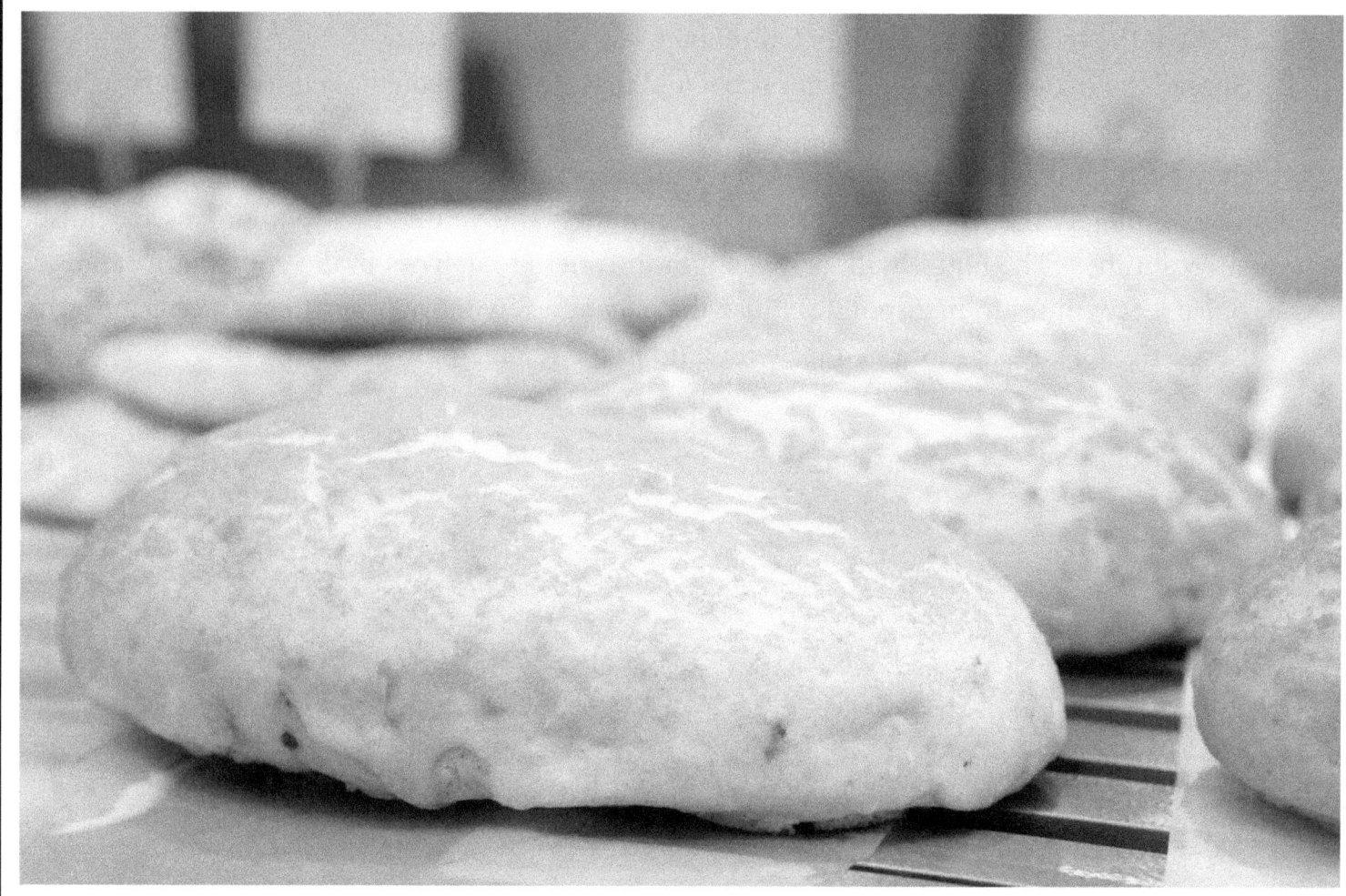

A delicious and unusual pumpkin bread. These little loaves are a hit with our household. Ideal for on-the-go munchies.

Nutrition

Calories: 368 | Protein: 8.5g | Fat: 12.7g | Cholesterol: 123.8mg | Sodium 427.3mg

Carbohydrates: 56.6g

Ingredients

Bread

- 3 eggs
- 1 ½ cups all-purpose flour
- 2 teaspoons pumpkin pie spice
- 2 cups canned pumpkin
- ½ cup white sugar
- 1 teaspoon baking soda
- ¾ cup brown sugar

Cream Cheese Filling

- 1 egg
- 2 teaspoons all-purpose flour
- 1 package cream cheese, softened to room temperature
- 4 tablespoons white sugar

Instructions

1. Preheat the oven to 350°F. Grease 8 tiny loaf pans, In the bowl of a stand mixer, combine the pumpkin and eggs and beat until smooth.
2. In a medium-sized mixing bowl, combine flour, brown sugar, white sugar, pumpkin spice, and baking soda. Pour into the pumpkin mixture and stir until it is completely smooth. Set aside.
3. In a mixing bowl, combine cream cheese, sugar, egg, and flour and beat until smooth.
4. Smooth out the cream cheese mixture evenly between the two pans. 1/2 of the pumpkin bread mixture must be poured or spooned evenly onto the bottom of each mini loaf pan. Over each cream cheese portion, pour the remaining bread mixture.
5. Bake for twenty-five to thirty minutes in a preheated oven or until a toothpick inserted in the center comes out clean. Allow for ten to fifteen minutes of resting time before serving.

CHOCOLATE ZUCCHINI BREAD

Preparation: 30 Minutes

Cook: 1 Hour

Servings: 20

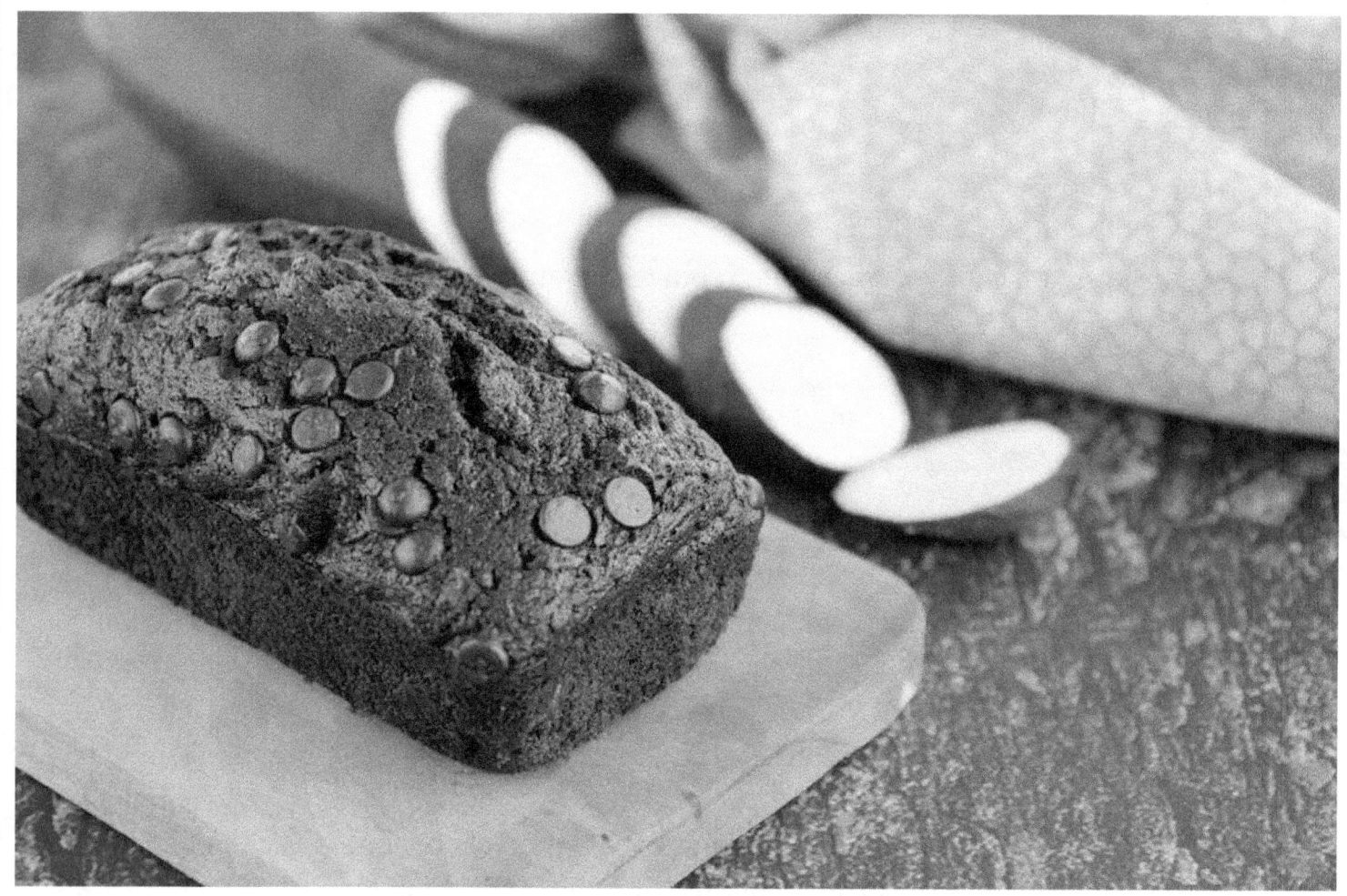

Even the kids will enjoy this moist, delicious bread with chocolate and spices. It's a fantastic way to use up all of your spare zucchinis from the garden!

Nutrition

Calories: 278 | Protein: 3g | Cholesterol: 27.9mg | Sodium: 192.6mg

Carbohydrates: 34.9g | Fat: 15.2g

Ingredients

- 2 cups grated zucchini
- 2 cups all-purpose flour
- 2 squares unsweetened chocolate
- 3 eggs
- 1 teaspoon ground cinnamon
- 2 cups white sugar
- 1 cup vegetable oil
- ¾ cup semisweet chocolate chips
- 1 teaspoon vanilla extract
- 1 teaspoon baking soda
- 1 teaspoon salt

Instructions

1. Preheat the oven to 350 degrees Fahrenheit. Grease two 9x5-inch loaf pans lightly. Microwave chocolate in a microwave-safe bowl until melted. Stir until the chocolate is completely smooth.
2. Combine eggs, sugar, oil, grated zucchini, vanilla, and chocolate in a large mixing dish and whisk thoroughly. Stir to combine baking soda, salt, and cinnamon in a mixing bowl. Mix the chocolate chips and fold them in. Pour the batter into the loaf pans that have been prepped.
3. Bake for sixty to seventy minutes in a preheated oven or until a toothpick inserted in the center of a loaf comes out clean.

LEMON PISTACHIO ZUCCHINI BREAD

Preparation: 25 Minutes

Cook: 45 Minutes

Servings: 20

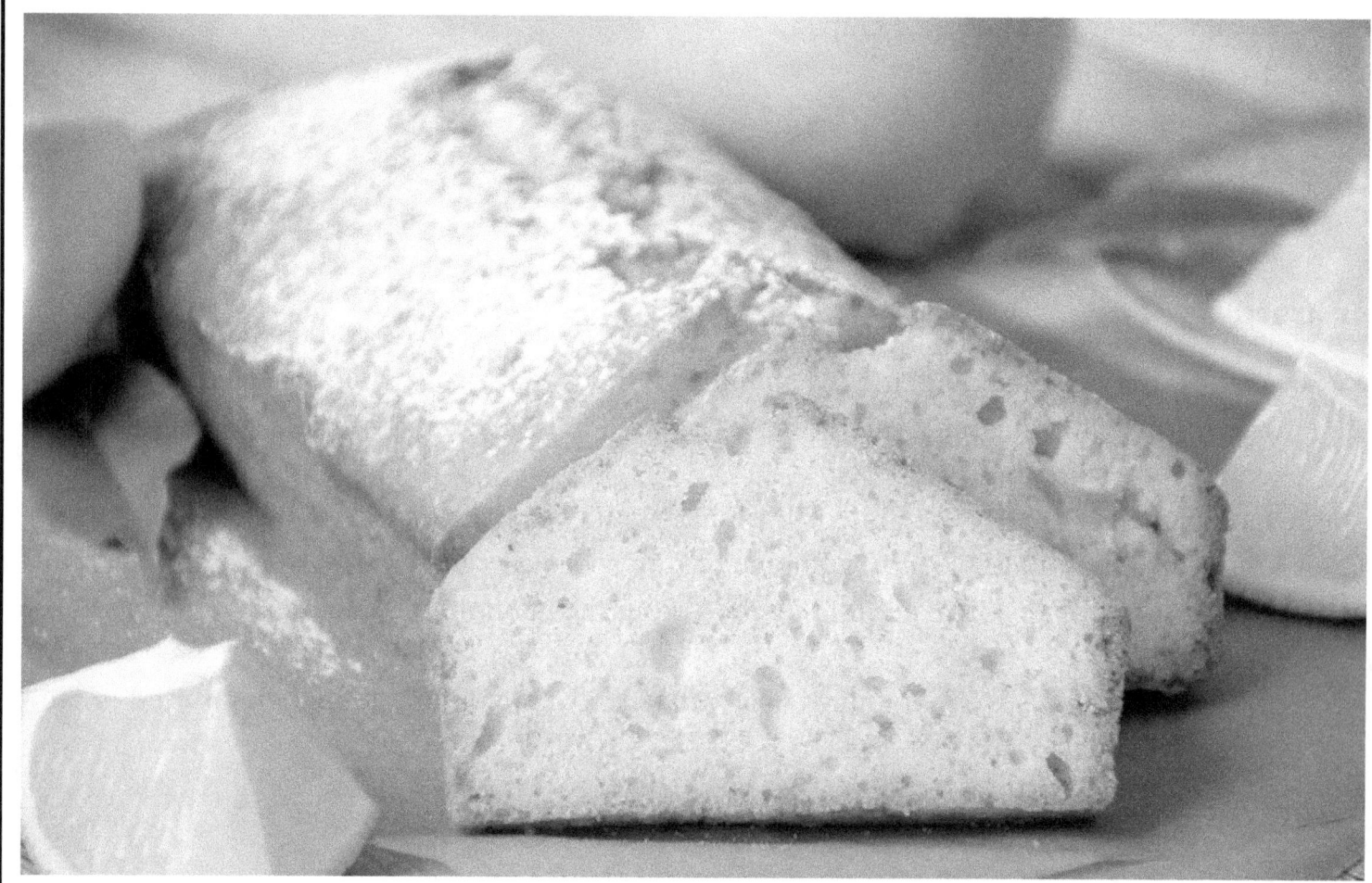

For a unique flavor, make moist zucchini bread with lemon and pistachios.

Nutrition

Calories: 293 | Protein: 5.3g | Cholesterol: 37.6mg | Sodium: 257.8mg

Carbohydrates: 34.5g | Fat: 15.3g

Ingredients

- cooking spray
- 4 eggs
- 1 ½ cups white sugar
- 1 cup vegetable oil
- 3 ½ cups all-purpose flour
- 1 tablespoon lemon juice
- 1 cup chopped pistachio nuts
- 1 ½ teaspoons baking soda
- 2 teaspoons vanilla extract
- 2 cups grated zucchini
- 1 teaspoon salt
- ½ cup plain yogurt
- 1 small lemon, zested

Instructions

1. Preheat the oven to 350 degrees Fahrenheit. Using cooking spray, coat two 9x5-inch loaf pans.
2. In a mixing bowl, combine flour, baking soda, and salt. In a separate dish, whisk together the eggs, sugar, and vegetable oil; toss in the yogurt, lemon zest, lemon juice, and vanilla essence. Stir the flour mixture into the wet ingredients until barely moistened, then fold in the zucchini and pistachios. Pour the batter evenly into the loaf pans that have been prepped.
3. Bake for forty-five to fifty-five minutes in a preheated oven or until a toothpick inserted in the center comes out clean. Cool for ten minutes in the pans before removing to a wire rack to cool fully.

BLUEBERRY ZUCCHINI BREAD

Preparation: 15 Minutes

Cook: 50 Minutes

Servings: 12

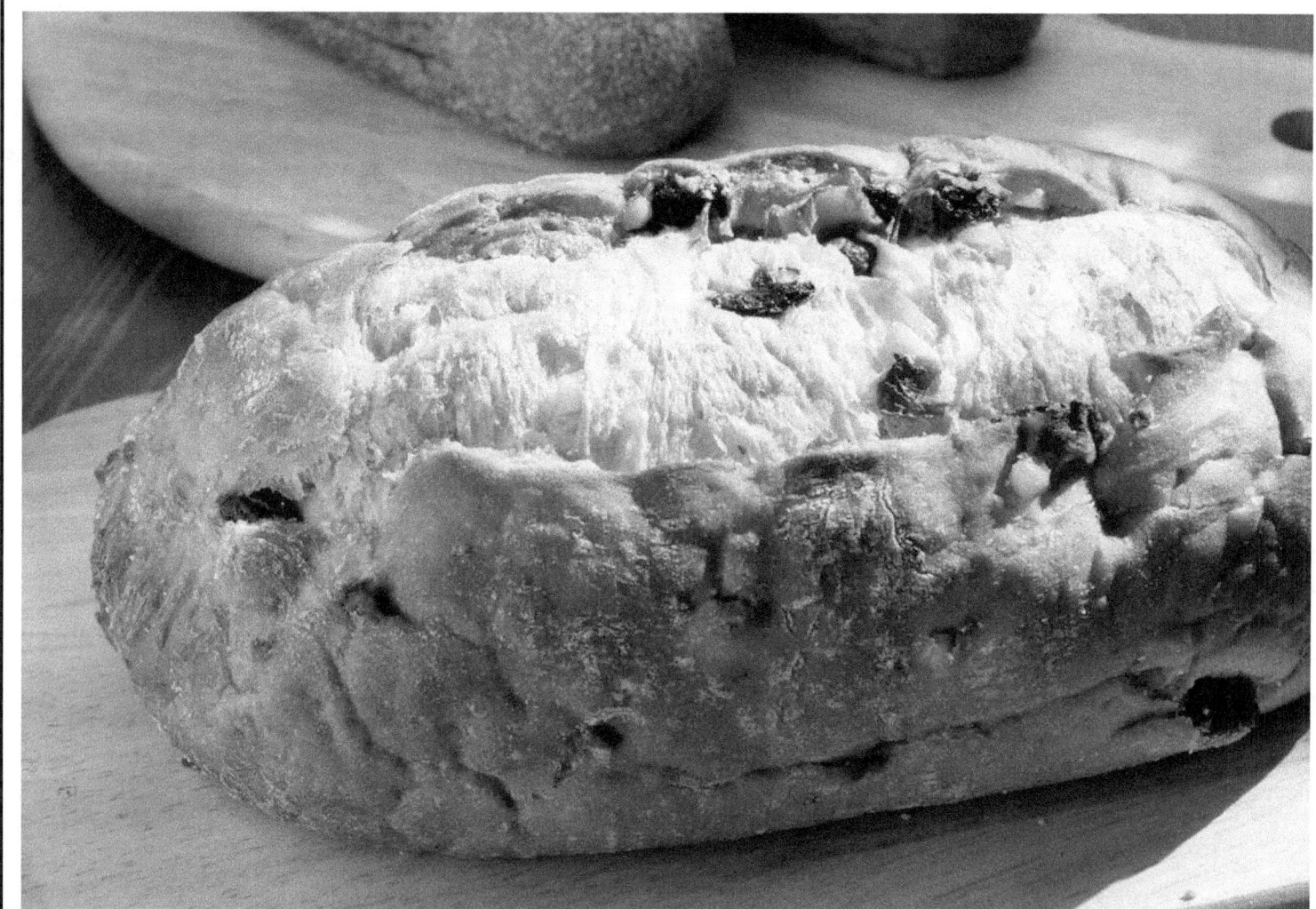

Blueberries and zucchini are made into delectable summer bread loaves.

Nutrition

Calories: 461 | Protein: 5.3g | Cholesterol: 46.5mg | Sodium: 281.3mg

Carbohydrates: 66.8g | Fat: 19.9g

Ingredients

- 2 cups shredded zucchini
- 3 cups all-purpose flour
- ¼ teaspoon baking soda
- 1 teaspoon baking powder
- 3 eggs, lightly beaten
- 1-pint fresh blueberries
- 1 tablespoon ground cinnamon
- 1 cup vegetable oil
- 2 ¼ cups white sugar
- 3 teaspoons vanilla extract
- 1 teaspoon salt

Instructions

1. Preheat the oven to 350 degrees Fahrenheit. Lightly grease 4 mini-loaf pans.
2. Mix the eggs, oil, vanilla, and sugar in a large mixing dish. Toss in the zucchini and mix well. Combine the flour, salt, baking powder, baking soda, and cinnamon in a large mixing bowl. Fold in the blueberries gently. Transfer to the mini-loaf pans that have been prepared.
3. Preheat oven to 350°F and bake for fifty minutes, or until a knife inserted in the center of a loaf comes out clean. Cool in pans for twenty minutes before turning out onto wire racks to cool fully.

ZUCCHINI BREAD WITH COCONUT

Preparation: 30 Minutes

Cook: 1 Hour

Servings: 8

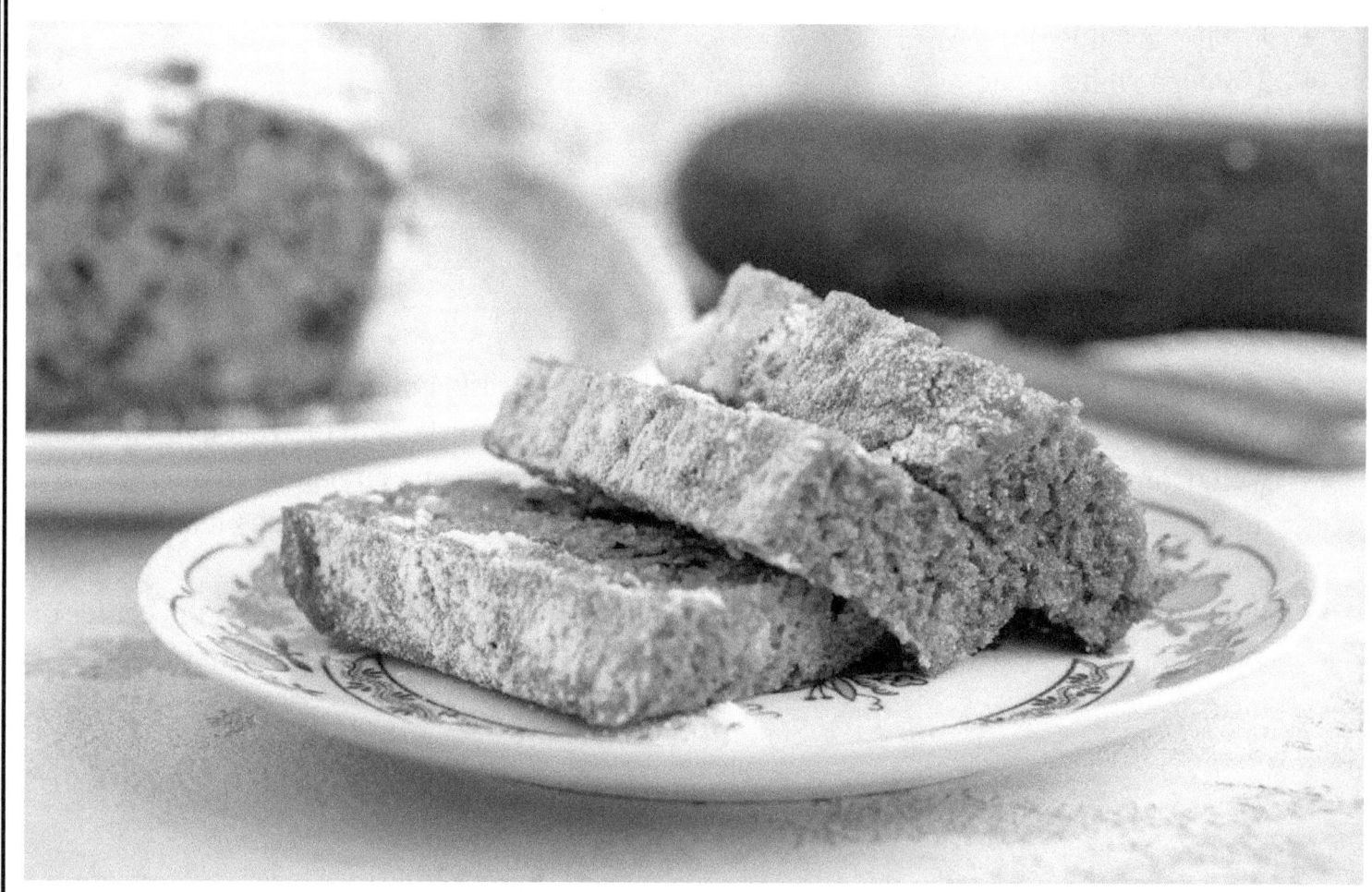

My favorite zucchini bread recipe, with a dash of coconut. After shredding the zucchini, squeeze out as much liquid as possible to avoid the cake becoming too mushy.

Nutrition

Calories: 574 | Protein: 7.5g | Cholesterol: 61.4mg | Sodium: 452.9mg

Carbohydrates: 67.6g | Fat: 31.9g

Ingredients

- 2 cups grated zucchini
- ¾ cup vegetable oil
- 2 teaspoons vanilla sugar
- 2 ½ cups all-purpose flour
- 1 ¼ cups unsweetened coconut flakes
- 1 teaspoon ground cinnamon
- 4 teaspoons baking powder
- 1 teaspoon baking soda
- 3 eggs, lightly beaten
- 1 pinch salt
- 1 ¼ cups white sugar

Instructions

1. Preheat the oven to 350 degrees Fahrenheit. Grease a loaf pan lightly.
2. In a mixing dish, combine flour, coconut, baking powder, baking soda, and salt.
3. In a second bowl, beat the sugar, oil, vanilla sugar, and cinnamon with an electric mixer until frothy.
4. Place grated zucchini in a sink colander. Squeeze out as much liquid as you can using your hands. Mix the zucchini and eggs into the sugar mixture thoroughly. Stir in the flour until everything is fully blended.
5. Pour the zucchini batter into the loaf pan that has been prepped.
6. Bake in the preheated oven for about one hour or until a toothpick inserted in the center of the cake comes out clean. Cool for ten minutes in the pan before inverting onto a wire rack to finish cooling.

PINEAPPLE COCONUT ZUCCHINI BREAD

Preparation: 30 Minutes

Cook: 50 Minutes

Servings: 24

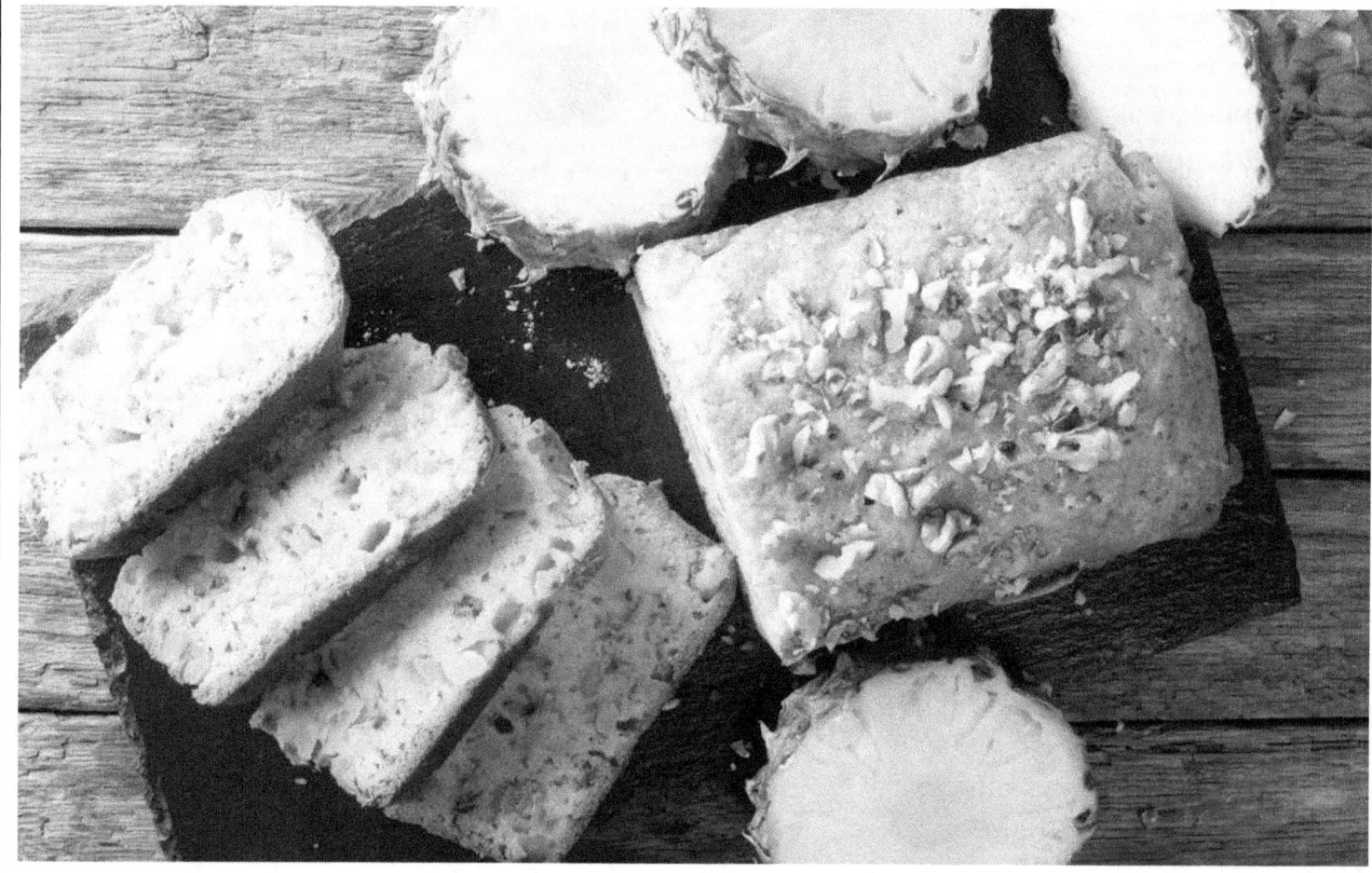

Zucchini bread is moist and tasty. This is a fantastic way to use up all of your zucchini from the garden.

Nutrition

Calories: 243 | Protein: 3g | Cholesterol: 25.4mg | Sodium: 248.1mg

Carbohydrates: 31.3g | Fat: 12.2g

Ingredients

- 3 eggs
- 1 cup vegetable oil
- 1 cup white sugar
- 3 cups grated unpeeled zucchini
- 3 cups all-purpose flour
- 1 cup light brown sugar
- ½ cup sour cream
- 2 teaspoons baking soda
- 1 teaspoon ground cinnamon
- 1 ½ teaspoons baking powder
- 2 teaspoons vanilla extract
- 1 teaspoon salt
- 1 teaspoon pumpkin pie spice
- 1 can crushed pineapple, well-drained
- ½ cup shredded coconut

Instructions

1. Preheat the oven to 350 degrees Fahrenheit. Grease two 9x5-inch loaf pans lightly. In a mixing bowl, combine flour, baking soda, baking powder, salt, cinnamon, and pumpkin pie spice; set aside.
2. In a large mixing bowl, whisk together the eggs, oil, white sugar, and brown sugar. Combine the sour cream, vanilla, zucchini, pineapple, and coconut in a mixing bowl. Mix in the flour mixture until it is just moistened. Divide the batter amongst the loaf pans that have been prepped.
3. Bake for fifty to sixty minutes, or until a toothpick inserted in the center comes out clean. Cool for ten minutes in the pans before removing and cooling completely on a wire rack.

BANANA-ZUCCHINI BREAD

Preparation: 15 Minutes

Cook: 50 Minutes

Servings: 20

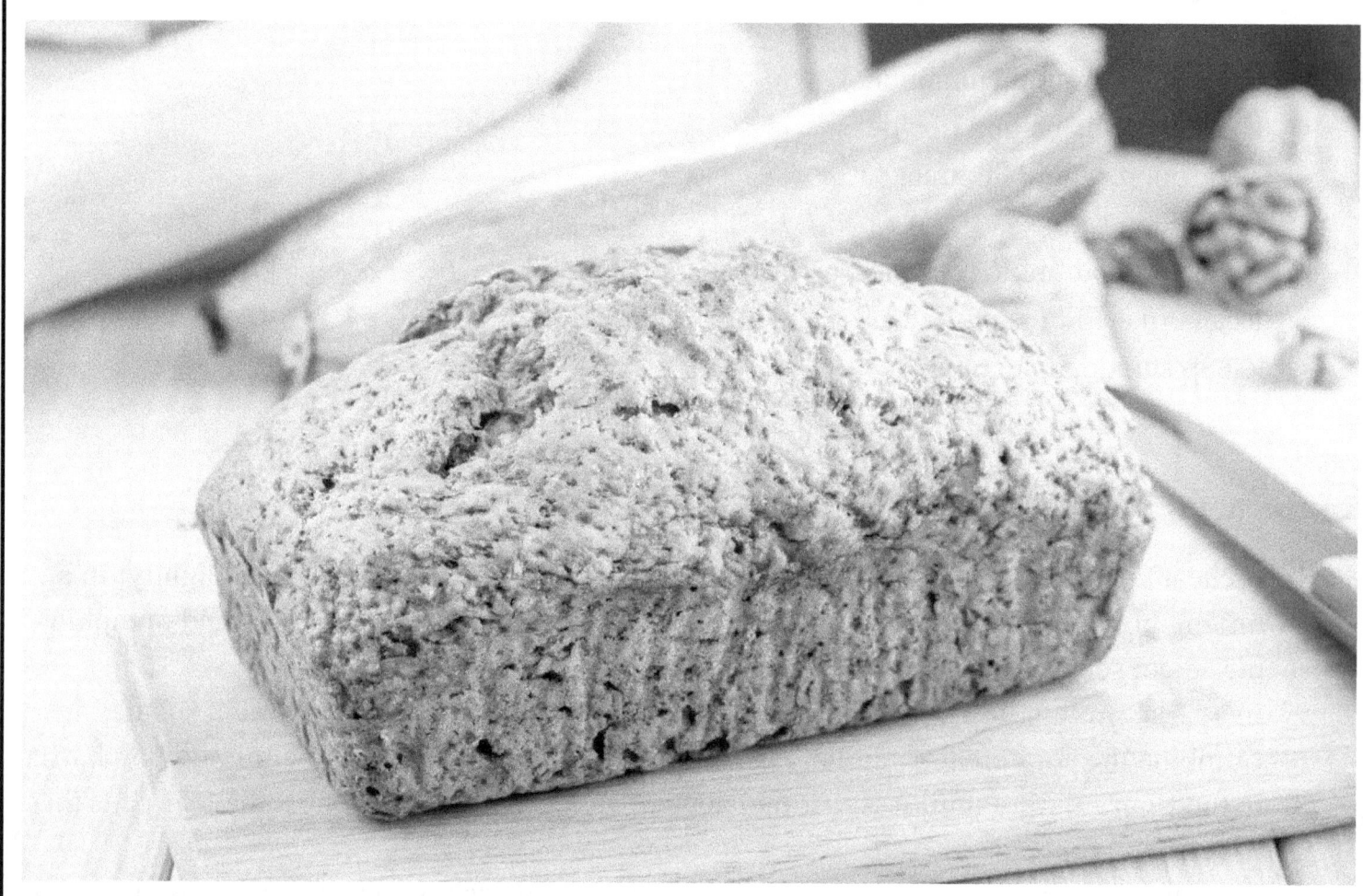

Banana nut bread and zucchini bread are combined in this recipe. The flavors blend together, leaving only a smidgeon of each flavor in each bite.

Nutrition

Calories: 272 | Protein: 3.9g | Cholesterol: 27.9mg | Sodium: 229.6mg

Carbohydrates: 40.2g | Fat: 11.1g

Ingredients

- 3 ½ cups all-purpose flour
- 2 teaspoons vanilla extract
- 1 tablespoon ground cinnamon
- ½ cup chopped walnuts
- ½ cup dried cranberries 3 eggs
- 1 ½ teaspoons baking powder
- ¾ cup vegetable oil
- 1 teaspoon baking soda
- 2 bananas, mashed
- ⅔ cup packed brown sugar
- 1 cup white sugar
- 1 cup grated zucchini
- 1 teaspoon salt

Instructions

1. Preheat the oven to 325°F. Two 8x4 inch bread loaf pans will be greased and floured.
2. In a large mixing dish, whisk the eggs until they are light yellow and foamy. Blend together the oil, brown sugar, white sugar, grated zucchini, bananas, and vanilla until completely blended. Combine the flour, cinnamon, baking powder, baking soda, and salt in a large mixing bowl.
3. Combine the cranberries and nuts in a mixing bowl. Divide the batter evenly between the two loaf pans that have been prepped.
4. Bake for fifty minutes in a preheated oven or until a toothpick inserted in the center comes out clean. Allow it to cool on a wire rack in the loaf pans before removing and serving.

ZUCCHINI APPLE BREAD

Preparation: 20 Minutes

Cook: 1 Hour

Servings: 24

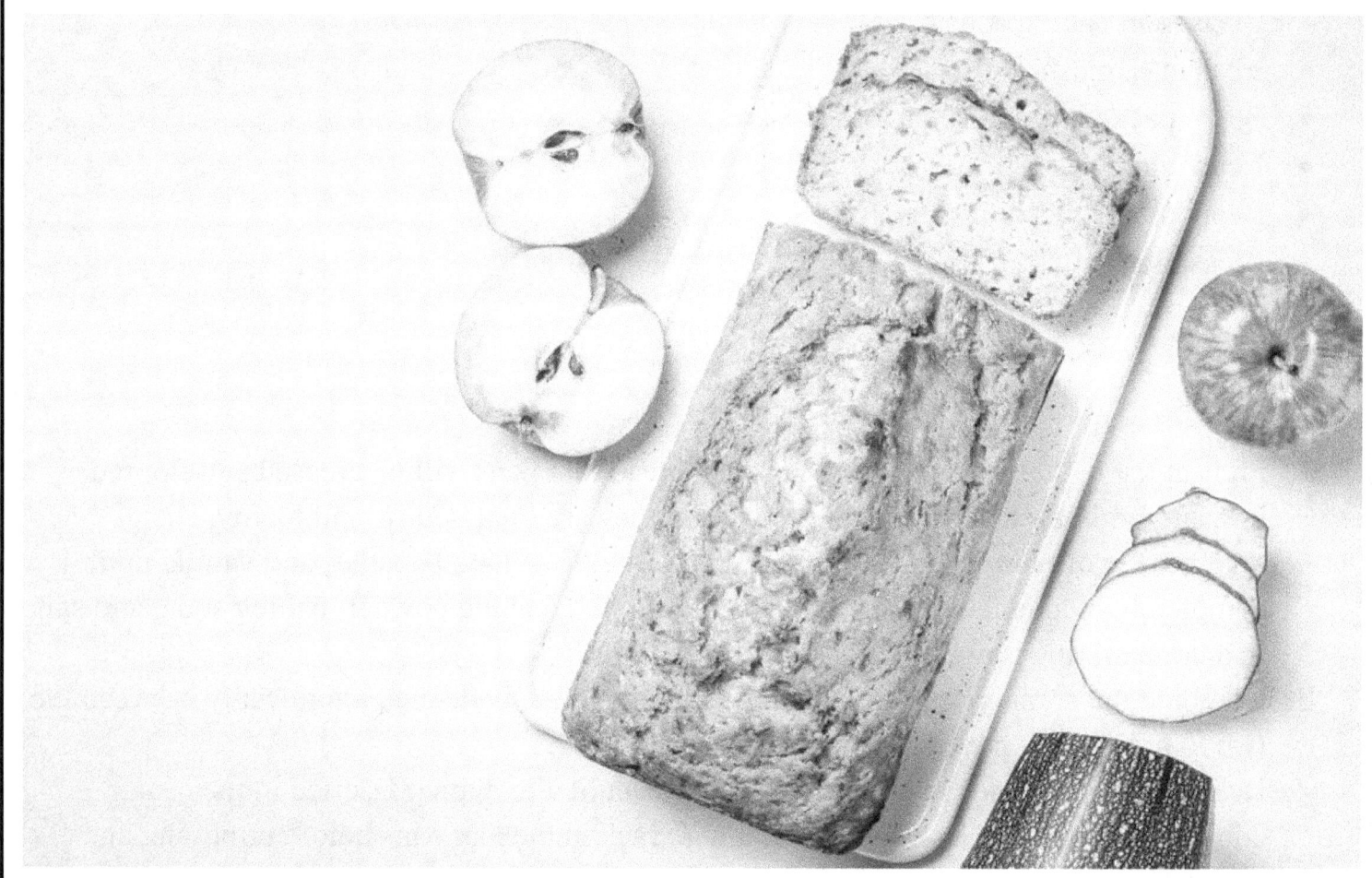

This zucchini bread version is fluffy and light, with a hint of sweetness.

Nutrition

Calories: 207 | Protein: 3.5g | Cholesterol: 31mg | Sodium: 142.9mg

Carbohydrates: 32.9g | Fat: 7.2g

Ingredients

- 3 ½ cups all-purpose flour
- 1 ½ teaspoons baking soda
- 2 cups peeled, chopped zucchini
- 1 teaspoon vanilla extract
- 2 teaspoons ground cinnamon
- 4 eggs
- ½ cup chopped walnuts
- 1 cup white sugar
- 1 cup brown sugar
- ½ cup vegetable oil
- ½ teaspoon salt
- 1 cup chopped, peeled apple

Instructions

1. Preheat the oven to 350 degrees Fahrenheit. Grease 2 - 9x5 inch loaf pans
2. Combine eggs, white sugar, brown sugar, oil, and vanilla in a large mixing bowl and whisk until thoroughly combined. Combine flour, baking soda, salt, and cinnamon in a separate bowl. In a separate bowl, whisk together the flour, baking powder, and salt. Mix walnuts, zucchini, and apple in a mixing bowl. Pour into the pans that have been prepared.
3. Bake for one hour or until the center of the top springs back when lightly touched. Allow ten minutes for cooling in pans before transferring to a wire rack to cool completely.

HARVEST VEGETABLE BREAD

Preparation: 25 Minutes

Cook: 55 Minutes

Servings: 10

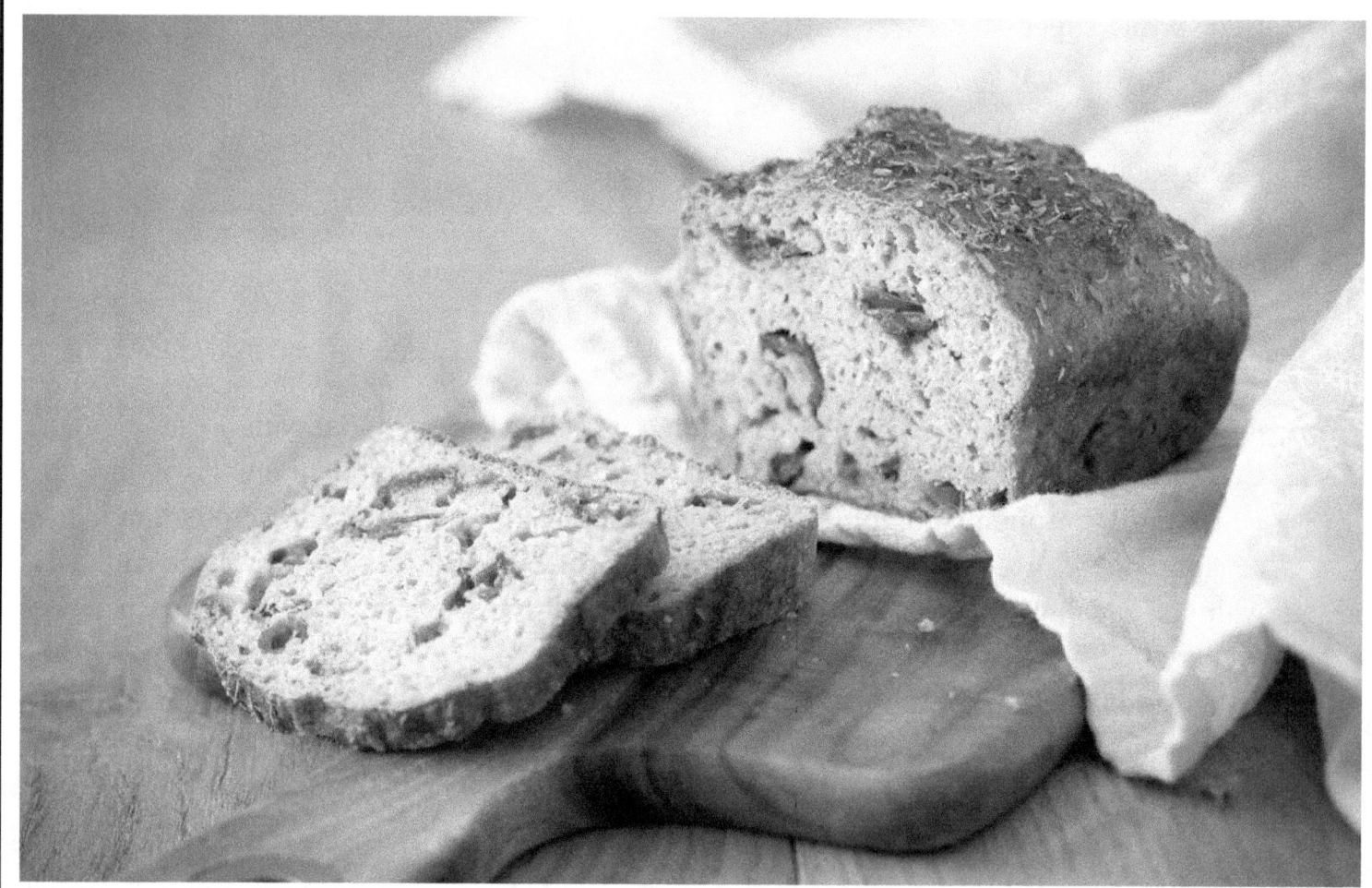

The perfect savory fast bread is made with garden-fresh zucchini, sun-dried tomatoes, and potatoes.

Nutrition

Calories: 207 | Protein: 3.5g | Cholesterol: 31mg | Sodium: 142.9mg

Carbohydrates: 32.9g | Fat: 7.2g

Ingredients

- ½ cup shredded parmesan cheese
- 3 ½ cups flour, plus extra for kneading
- ⅓ cup vegetable oil
- ⅓ cup sliced green onion tops
- 1 cup mashed potatoes
- ¾ cup Almond Breeze Original Unsweetened almond milk
- ½ teaspoon salt
- 1 egg
- ¾ cup shredded zucchini
- ⅓ cup minced sun-dried tomato
- 1 ½ tablespoons baking powder

Instructions

1. Preheat the oven to 375 degrees F and gently grease or parchment paper on a baking sheet.
2. Mix mashed potatoes, Almond Breeze, oil, and egg in a large mixing bowl until well combined. Stir zucchini, sun-dried tomatoes, and green onions in a mixing bowl. In a medium bowl and mix, combine the remaining ingredients and whisk them into the vegetable mixture.
3. Knead the dough several times on a floured surface until it is smooth. Form into a loaf and place on a baking pan lined with parchment paper.
4. Preheat oven to 350°F and bake for fifty-five minutes, or until a toothpick inserted in the middle comes out clean.

HEARTY BREAKFAST MUFFINS

Preparation: 20 Minutes

Cook: 20 Minutes

Servings: 12

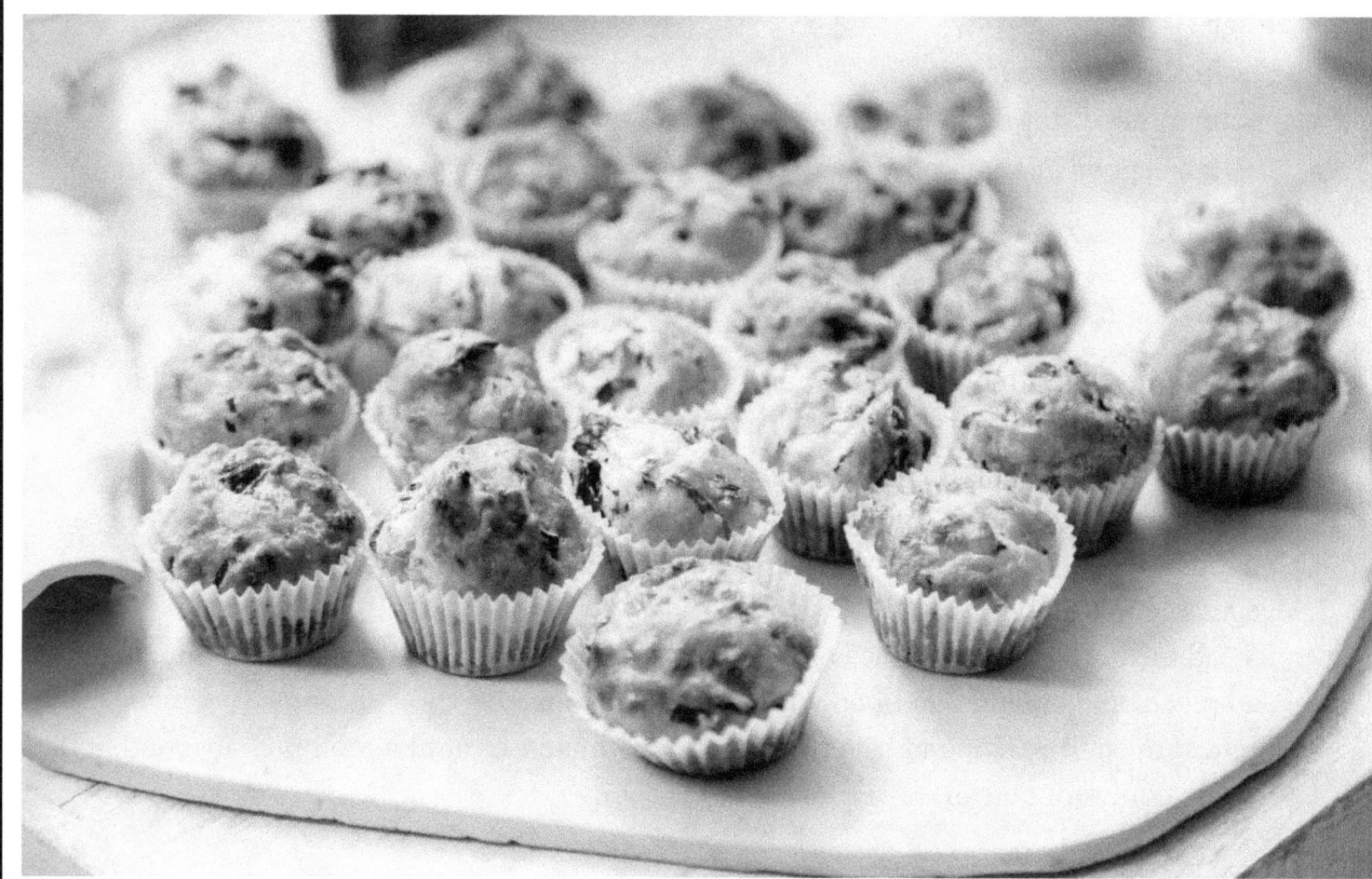

Breakfast muffins that are both healthy and filling. These have a mild sweetness to them and many healthy nutrients to help you start your day. Moisturizing, chewy, and not too dense. It's really adaptable! You can use any type of yogurt, but plain Greek yogurt is preferred. Add your favorite nuts or seeds, zucchini or squash, cooked sweet potato, raisins or cranberries, and so on to make it your own. Enjoy

Nutrition

Calories: 227 | Protein: 4.5g | Cholesterol: 31.3mg | Sodium: 388.1mg

Carbohydrates: 31.7g | Fat: 10.1g

Ingredients

- 2 eggs
- ½ cup shredded coconut
- ½ cup rolled oats
- 1 cup whole wheat flour
- ½ teaspoon ground ginger 2 carrots, shredded
- 1 teaspoon ground cinnamon
- 1 ½ teaspoons baking soda
- 2 bananas, mashed
- ½ cup packed brown sugar
- 1 zucchini, shredded
- ¼ cup vegetable oil
- ½ cup chopped pecans
- ½ cup dried cherries
- ¼ cup yogurt
- 1 teaspoon salt

Instructions

1. Preheat the oven to 375 degrees Fahrenheit. Grease 12 muffin cups or line with paper liners
2. Combine carrots, banana, zucchini, vegetable oil, yogurt, and eggs in a mixing bowl until well mixed.
3. In a separate bowl, combine the flour and baking soda. Brown sugar, oats, coconut, pecans, cherries, cinnamon, salt, and ginger must all be incorporated into the flour mixture. Combine wet and dry ingredients in a mixing bowl and stir until just blended. Scoop the batter into the muffin cups that have been prepared.
4. Bake until a toothpick inserted in the center of a muffin comes out clean, and the sides are slightly golden, seventeen to twenty-two minutes in a preheated oven. Cool for ten minutes in the pans before removing to a wire rack to cool fully.

SAVORY CHEDDAR ZUCCHINI MUFFINS

Preparation: 20 Minutes

Cook: 1 Hour

Servings: 24

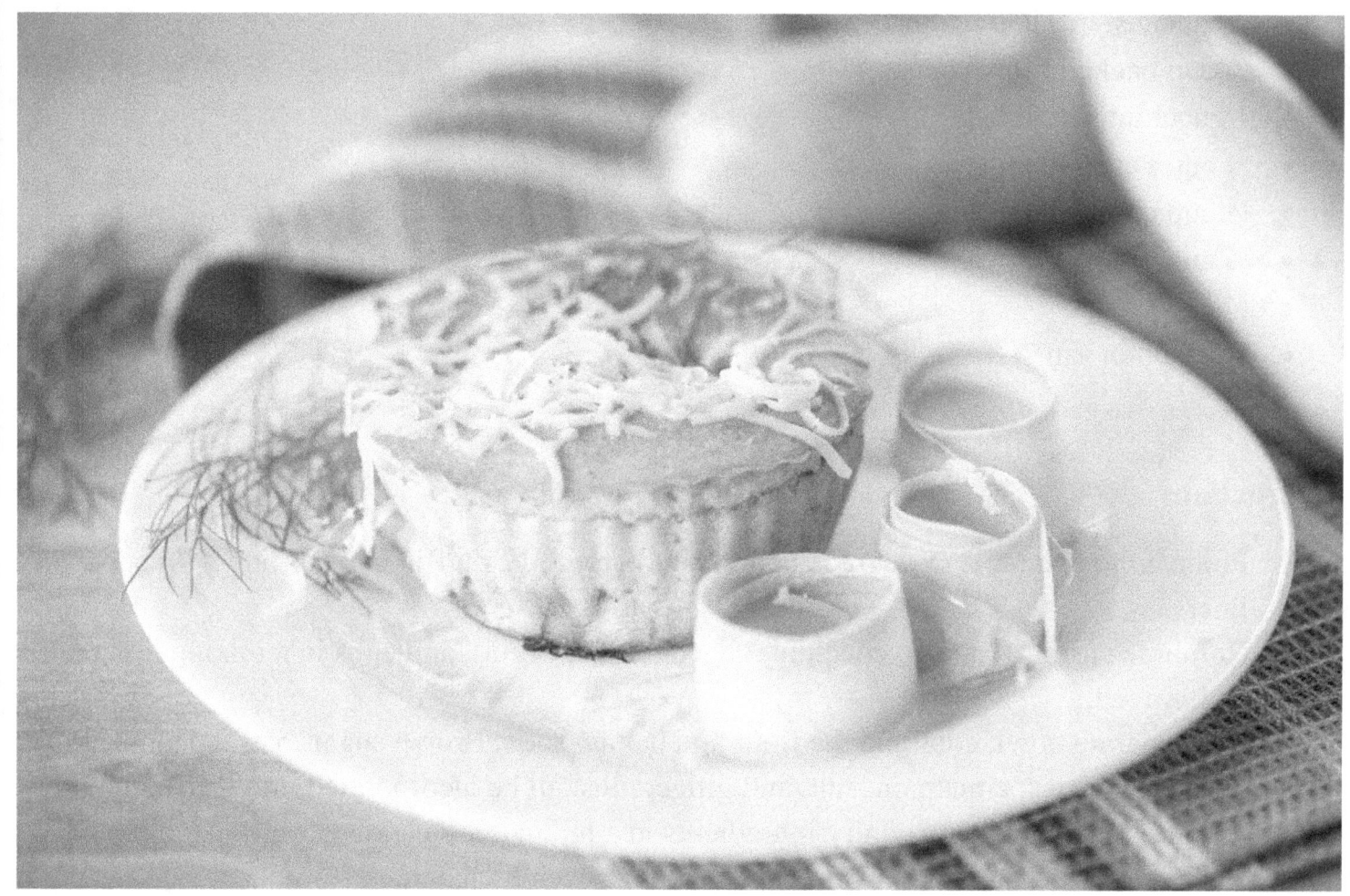

These savory muffins are also excellent for a quick breakfast! Even people who think they don't like zucchini love them!

Nutrition

Calories: 255 | Protein: 3.3g | Cholesterol: 23.3mg | Sodium: 179.8mg

Carbohydrates: 32.1g | Fat: 13.1g

Ingredients

- ¼ cup butter, melted
- ¼ cup freshly grated Parmesan cheese
- ½ teaspoon salt
- ¾ cup shredded Cheddar cheese
- 1 clove garlic, minced
- 1 cup milk
- 1 cup shredded unpeeled zucchini
- 1 egg, lightly beaten
- 1 teaspoon baking soda
- 1 ½ teaspoons baking powder
- 1 ¾ cups all-purpose flour
- 4 slices bacon, cooked crisp and crumbled

Instructions

1. Preheat the oven to 350 degrees Fahrenheit. Using cooking spray, coat 12 muffin cups.
2. In a mixing bowl, combine the flour, baking powder, baking soda, and salt.
3. In a separate bowl, thoroughly combine the butter, egg, milk, zucchini, and garlic. Mix about 1/2 cup of the flour mixture into the milk mixture at a time, stirring after each addition, until the flour mixture is fully integrated. Pour the batter into the prepared muffin cups, folding in the Cheddar cheese, Parmesan cheese, and crumbled bacon.
4. Bake for thirty to thirty-five minutes, or until a toothpick inserted in the center of a muffin comes out clean. Remove muffins from muffin cups and set aside to cool slightly before serving warm. Keep leftovers refrigerated.

KINGMAN'S VEGAN ZUCCHINI BREAD

Preparation: 20 Minutes

Cook: 1 Hour 10 Minutes

Servings: 24

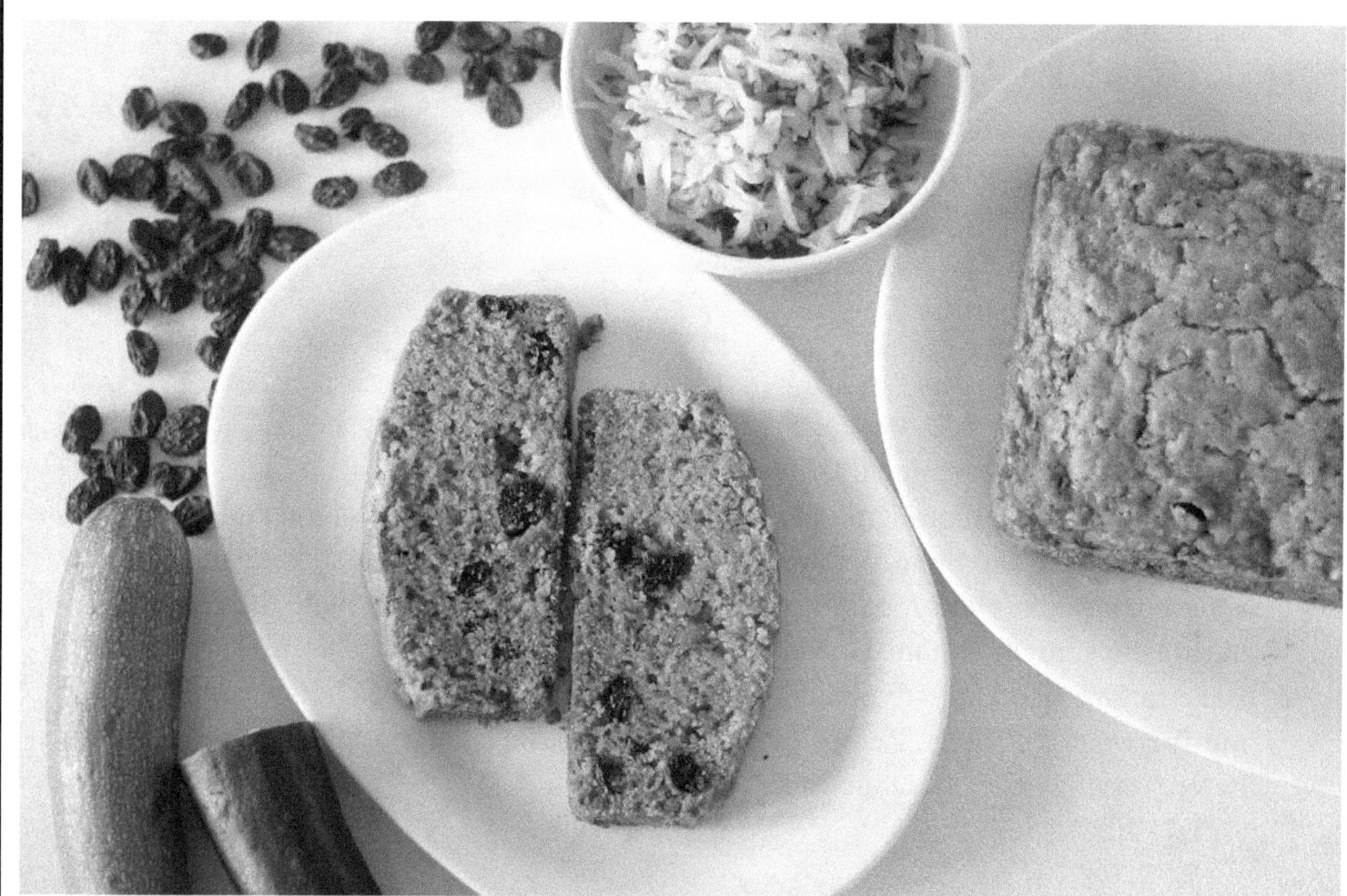

Delicious. Fluffy. Mm-hmmm.

Nutrition

Calories: 200 | Protein: 2.1g | Fat: 7.6g | Sodium: 164.4mg | Carbohydrates: 31.5g

Ingredients

- ½ teaspoon baking powder
- ¾ cup vegetable oil
- 1 cup packed brown sugar
- 1 cup unsweetened applesauce
- 1 cup white sugar
- 1 teaspoon baking soda
- 1 teaspoon salt
- 2 teaspoons ground cinnamon
- 2 teaspoons vanilla extract
- 2 ½ cups shredded zucchini
- 3 cups all-purpose flour
- 3 tablespoons flax seeds (Optional)
- ½ teaspoon arrowroot powder (Optional)

Instructions

1. Preheat the oven to 325°F. Grease 2 9x5 inch loaf pans and flour. In a mixing bowl, combine the flour, flax seeds, salt, baking soda, cinnamon, baking powder, and arrowroot until well combined; set aside.
2. In a large mixing bowl, combine the applesauce, white sugar, brown sugar, vegetable oil, and vanilla extract until smooth. Mix in the flour and shredded zucchini until everything is moistened. Divide the batter amongst the loaf pans that have been prepped.
3. Bake for seventy minutes in a preheated oven or until a toothpick inserted in the center comes out clean. Cool for ten minutes in the pans before removing to a wire rack to cool fully.

JALAPENO GREEN ONION ALE CORN BREAD

Preparation: 10 Minutes

Cook: 30 Minutes

Servings: 8

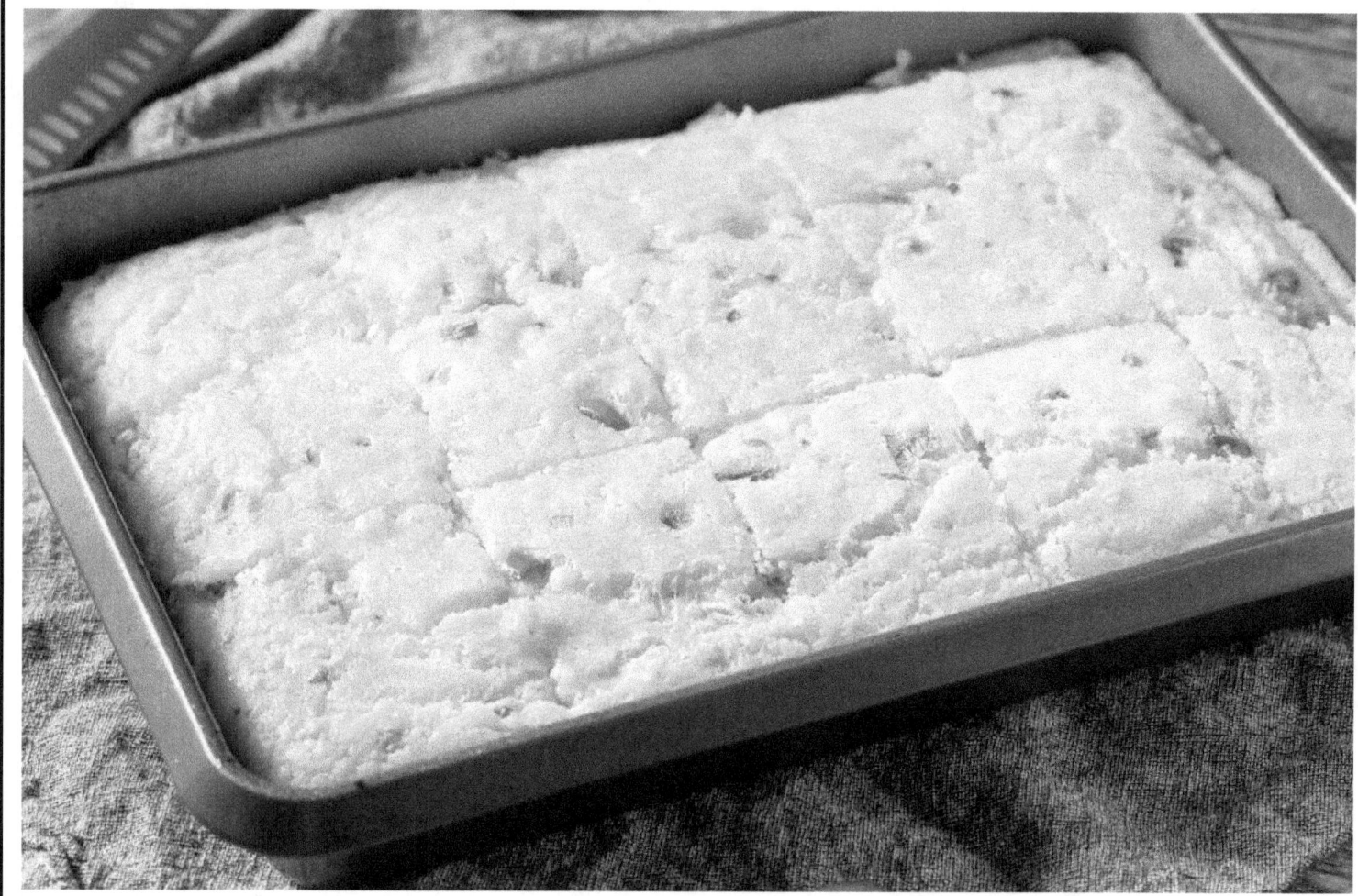

This sweet and spicy corn bread goes great with grilled cuisine or a Mexican supper.

Nutrition

Calories: 289 | Protein: 5.3g | Cholesterol: 77.6mg | Sodium: 627.6mg

Carbohydrates: 36.1g | Fat: 13.4g

Ingredients

- ⅓ cup white sugar
- ½ cup beer
- ½ cup butter, melted
- ½ cup buttermilk
- 1 cup all-purpose flour
- 1 cup cornmeal
- 1 fresh jalapeno pepper, chopped
- 1 teaspoon baking powder
- 1 teaspoon baking soda
- 1 teaspoon salt
- 2 eggs, beaten
- 4 green onions, chopped

Instructions

1. Preheat the oven to 400 degrees Fahrenheit. Grease a loaf pan and set it aside.
2. In a large mixing bowl, combine cornmeal, flour, baking powder, baking soda, and salt.
3. In a separate dish, combine the buttermilk, beer, and melted butter; gradually whisk into the cornmeal mixture to form a batter. Stir in the eggs and sugar to the batter. Mix in the green onions and jalapeño pepper, then pour into the prepared loaf pan.
4. Bake thirty to thirty-five minutes in a preheated oven until a knife inserted in the center comes out clean. Cool for ten minutes in the pan before removing to a wire rack to cool fully.

SWEET CORN CAKE

Preparation: 15 Minutes

Cook: 1Hour

Servings: 6

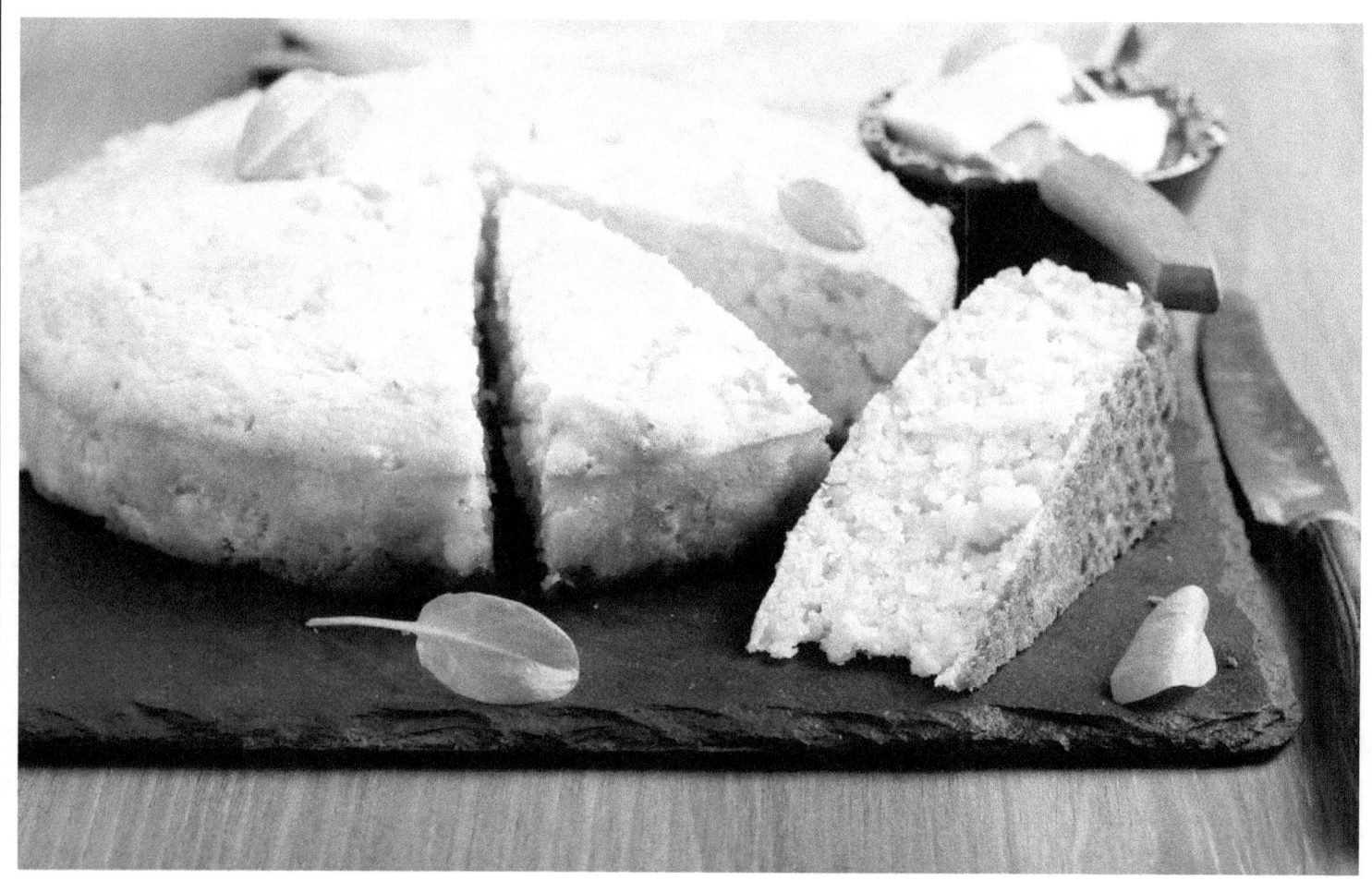

A sweet corn cake with a spoon bread consistency from Mexico.

Nutrition

Calories: 273 | Protein: 2.6g | Cholesterol: 47.5mg | Sodium: 256.9mg

Carbohydrates: 27.9g | Fat: 18.1g

Ingredients

- ¼ cup cornmeal
- ¼ cup water
- ¼ teaspoon salt
- ⅓ cup white sugar
- ⅓ cup masa harina
- ½ cup butter softened
- ½ teaspoon baking powder
- 1 ½ cups frozen whole-kernel corn, thawed
- 2 tablespoons heavy whipping cream

Instructions

1. Process thawed corn in a food processor, but keep it chunky. Incorporate the flour into the butter mixture.
2. In a medium mixing bowl, cream the butter. Mix in the Mexican cornflour and water until thoroughly combined.
3. Combine cornmeal, sugar, cream, salt, and baking powder in a separate bowl. Stir in the cornflour mixture until everything is well combined. Pour the batter into an 8x8 inch baking pan that hasn't been buttered. Cover with aluminum foil and smooth up the batter. Place the pan in a 9x13 inch baking dish that is half-filled with water.
4. Preheat the oven to 350 degrees F and bake for fifty to sixty minutes. Allow ten minutes for cooling. For easy removal from the pan, use an ice cream scoop.

HONEY CORNBREAD

Preparation: 8 Minutes

Cook: 25 Minutes

Servings: 8

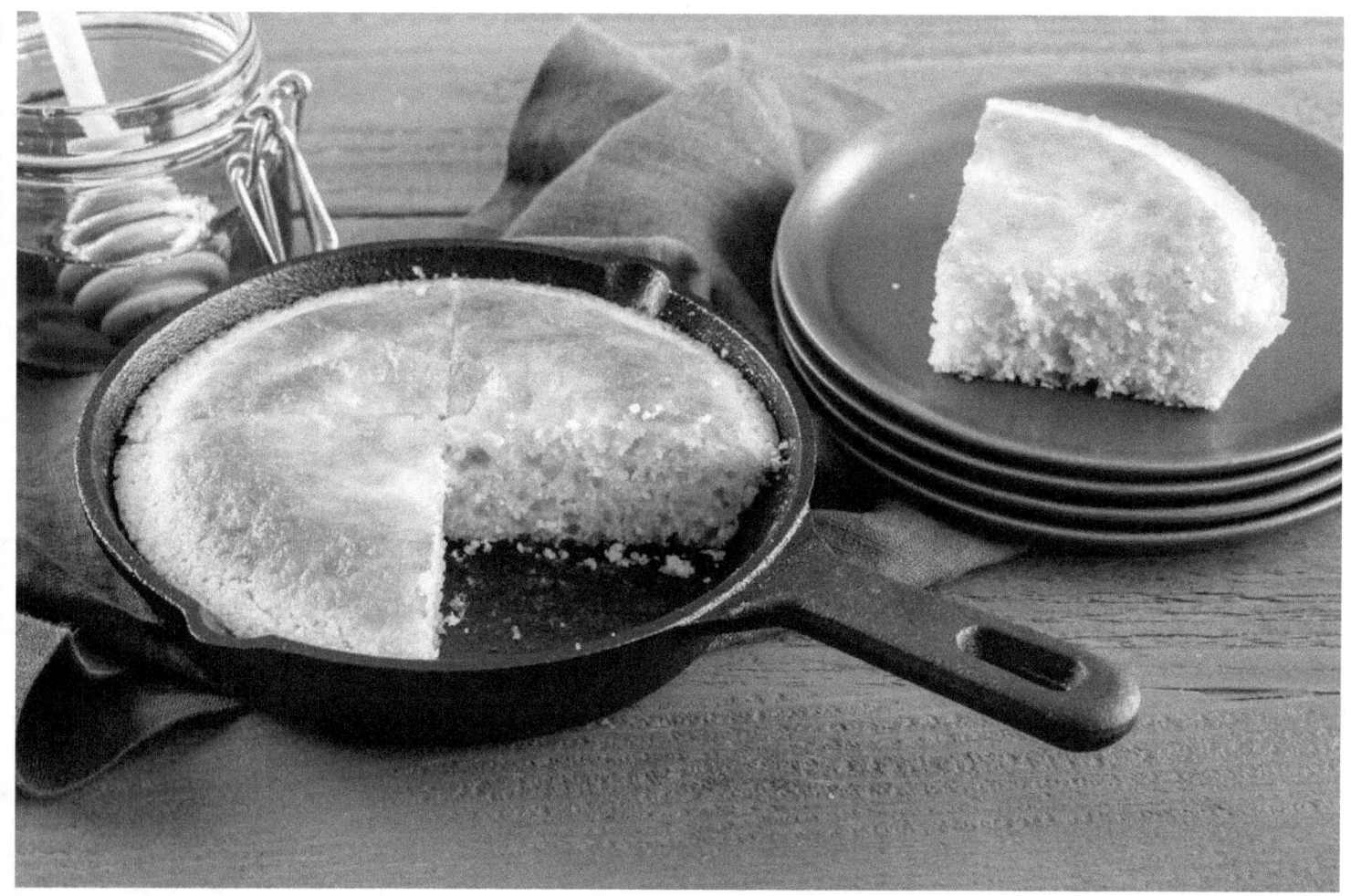

This sweet cornbread crumbles in your hands and melts in your mouth.

Nutrition

Calories: 358 | Protein: 5.1g | Cholesterol: 87.3mg | Sodium: 156.6mg

Carbohydrates: 41.8g | Fat: 19.5g

Ingredients

- ¼ cup honey
- ¼ cup vegetable oil
- ¼ cup white sugar
- 1 cup all-purpose flour
- 1 cup heavy cream
- 1 cup yellow cornmeal
- 1 tablespoon baking powder
- 2 eggs, lightly beaten

Instructions

1. Preheat the oven to 400 degrees Fahrenheit. Grease a 9x9-inch baking pan lightly.
2. Combine flour, cornmeal, sugar, and baking powder in a large mixing bowl. In the center of the dry ingredients, make a well. Combine the cream, oil, honey, and eggs in a mixing bowl. Pour the batter into the baking pan that has been prepared.
3. Bake for twenty to twenty-five minutes in a preheated oven or until a toothpick inserted in the center of the pan comes out clean.

BLUEBERRY CORNBREAD

Preparation: 15 Minutes

Cook: 25 Minutes

Servings: 6

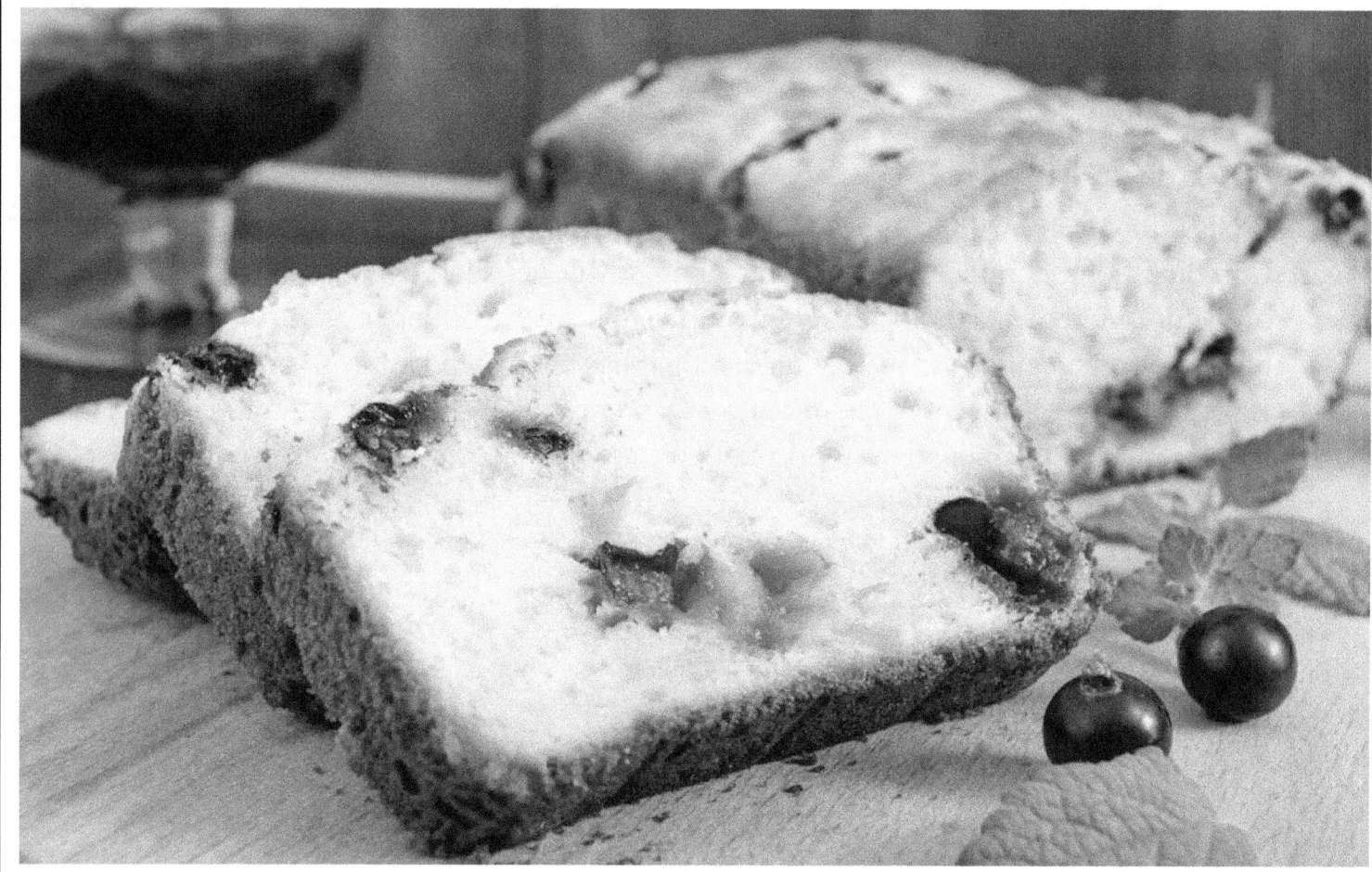

Cornbread cooked from scratch with wonderful blueberries. This is a fantastic mix! Blueberries can be used fresh or frozen.

Nutrition

Calories: 453 | Protein: 7.2g | Cholesterol: 64.2mg | Sodium: 668.3mg

Carbohydrates: 59.8g | Fat: 21.3g

Ingredients

- ½ cup vegetable oil
- ½ cup white sugar
- ⅔ cup milk
- 1 cup all-purpose flour
- 1 cup cornmeal
- 1 teaspoon salt
- 2 cups blueberries
- 2 eggs
- 3 teaspoons baking powder

Instructions

1. Preheat the oven to 400 degrees Fahrenheit. A 9-inch square baking dish should be greased.
2. In a mixing bowl, mix cornmeal, flour, sugar, baking powder, and salt. In a separate large mixing bowl, whisk together the eggs, milk, and oil. Combine the cornmeal and egg mixture and stir until barely mixed. Fold blueberries into the mixture and pour into the baking dish that has been prepared.
3. Bake for twenty-five to thirty minutes in a preheated oven, or until a toothpick inserted in the center comes out clean.

ABSOLUTE MEXICAN CORNBREAD

Preparation: 15 Minutes

Cook: 1 Hour

Servings: 6

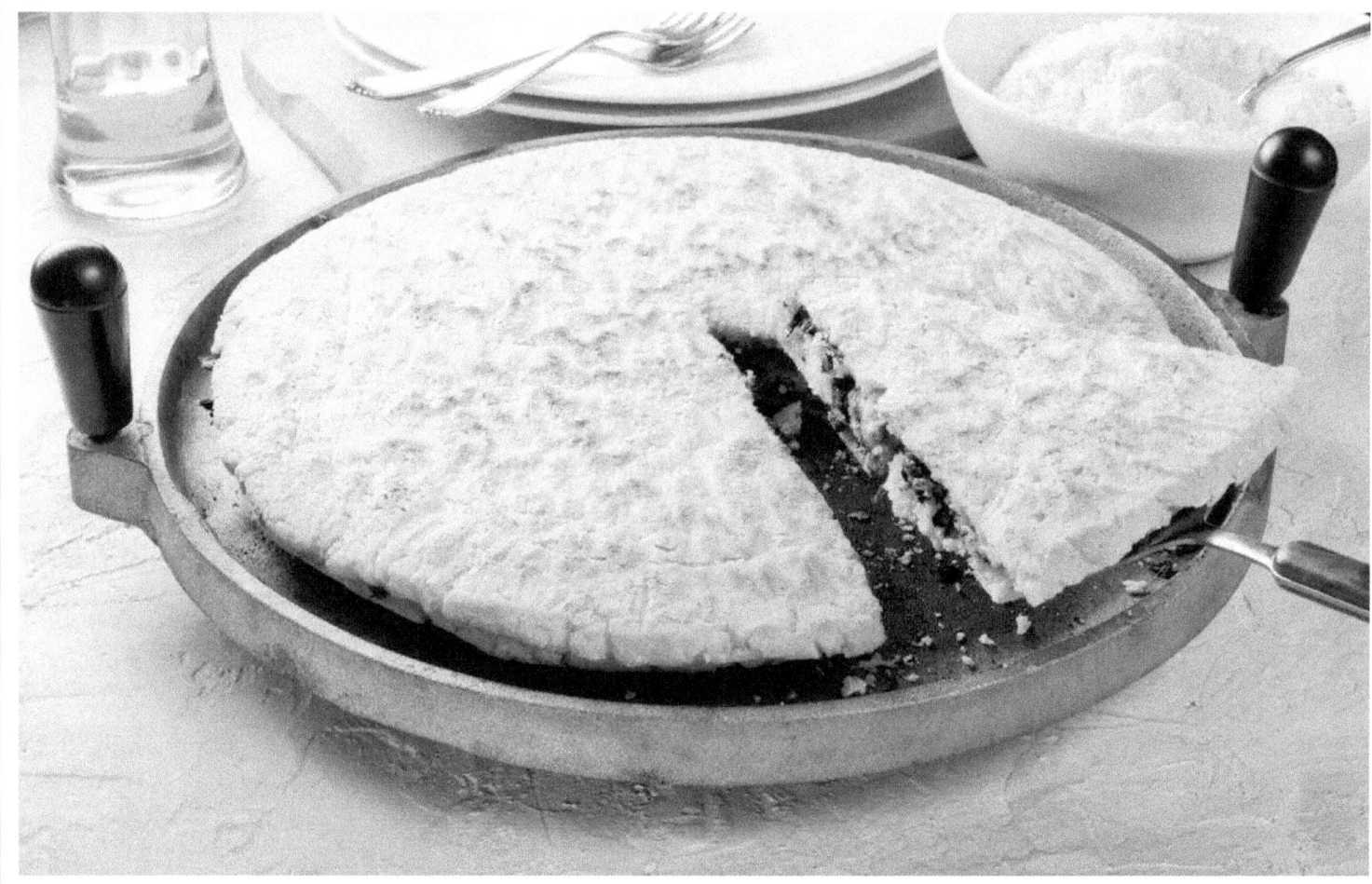

This has to be the most delicious and moist cornbread we've ever made. It is the most often requested item. Don't be fooled by the ingredients. It's incredible.

Nutrition

Calories: 743 | Protein: 14.5g | Cholesterol: 223.6mg | Sodium: 1050.7mg

Carbohydrates: 83.6g | Fat: 40.9g

Ingredients

- ¼ teaspoon salt
- ½ can of chopped green chile peppers, drained
- ½ cup shredded Cheddar cheese
- ½ cup shredded Monterey Jack cheese
- can cream-style corn
- 1 cup all-purpose flour
- 1 cup butter, melted
- 1 cup white sugar
- 1 cup yellow cornmeal
- 4 eggs
- 4 teaspoons baking powder

Instructions

1. Preheat the oven to 300 degrees Fahrenheit. Grease a 9x13-inch baking dish lightly.
2. Butter and sugar must be combined in a large mixing dish. One at a time beat in the eggs. Mix cream corn, chiles, Monterey Jack, and Cheddar cheeses in a mixing bowl.
3. Combine flour, cornmeal, baking powder, and salt in a separate bowl. Stir the flour mixture into the corn mixture until it is completely smooth. Pour the batter into the pan that has been prepared.
4. Bake for one hour in a preheated oven or until a toothpick inserted in the center comes out clean.

EXCELLENT AND HEALTHY CORNBREAD

Preparation: 10 Minutes

Cook: 25 Minutes

Servings: 12

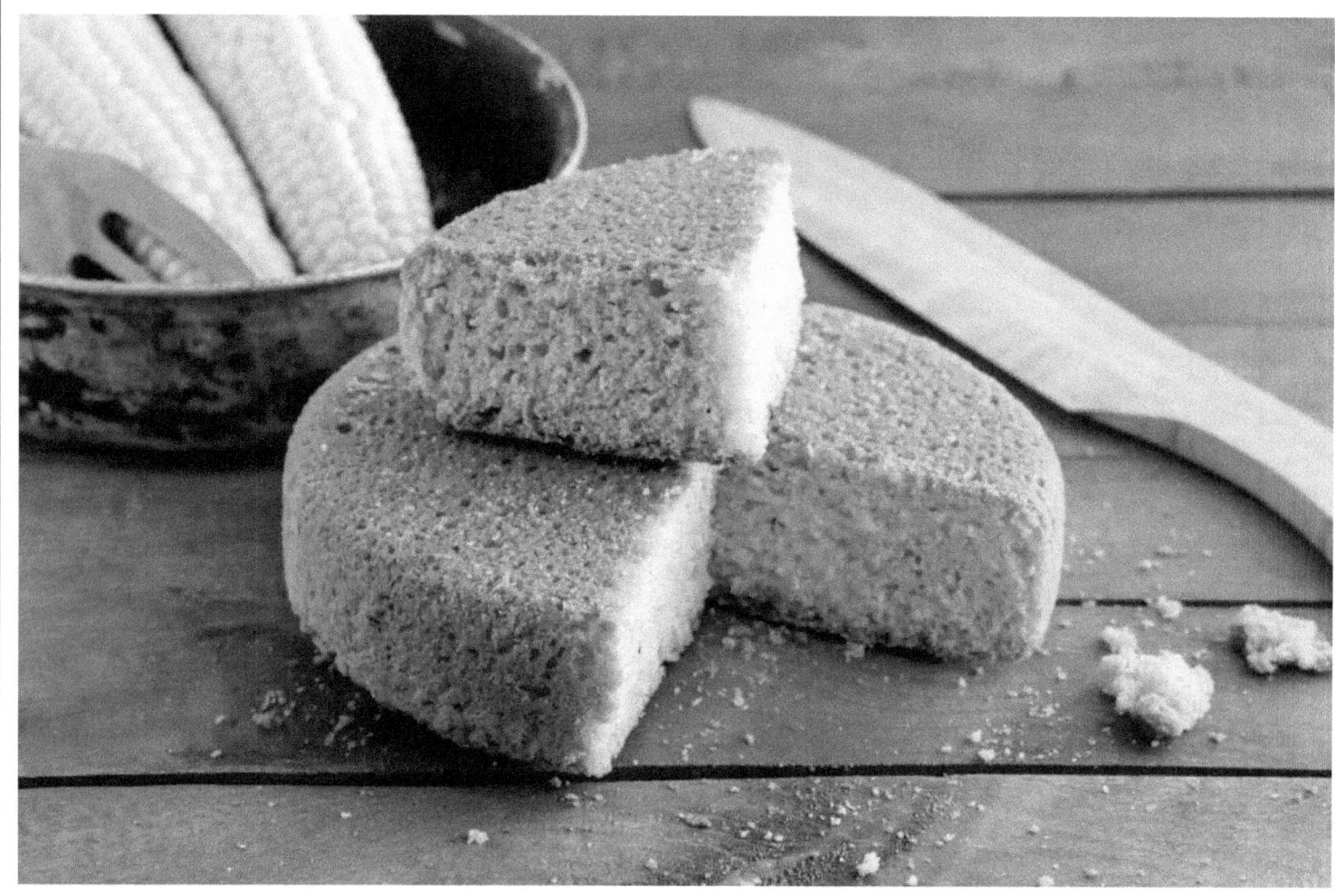

This cornbread recipe requires no oil and tastes fantastic. Serve with honey, butter, or margarine while still warm.

Nutrition

Calories: 76 | Protein: 3g | Cholesterol: 31.4mg | Sodium: 281.2mg

Carbohydrates: 13.6g | Fat: 1.2g

Ingredients

- ¼ cup white sugar
- ¾ teaspoon salt
- 1 cup cornmeal
- 1 cup plain nonfat yogurt
- 1 cup unbleached flour
- 1 teaspoon baking soda
- 2 eggs, beaten

Instructions

1. Preheat the oven to 400 degrees Fahrenheit. Grease an 8x8 inch baking pan lightly.
2. Combine flour, cornmeal, sugar, soda, and salt in a large mixing dish. Stir the yogurt and eggs in a mixing bowl. Don't overmix; merely stir until everything is fully combined. Pour the batter into the pan that has been prepared.
3. Bake for twenty to twenty-five minutes in a preheated oven or until the bread springs back when lightly pressed in the center.

GOLDEN SWEET CORNBREAD

Preparation: 10 Minutes

Cook: 25 Minutes

Servings: 12

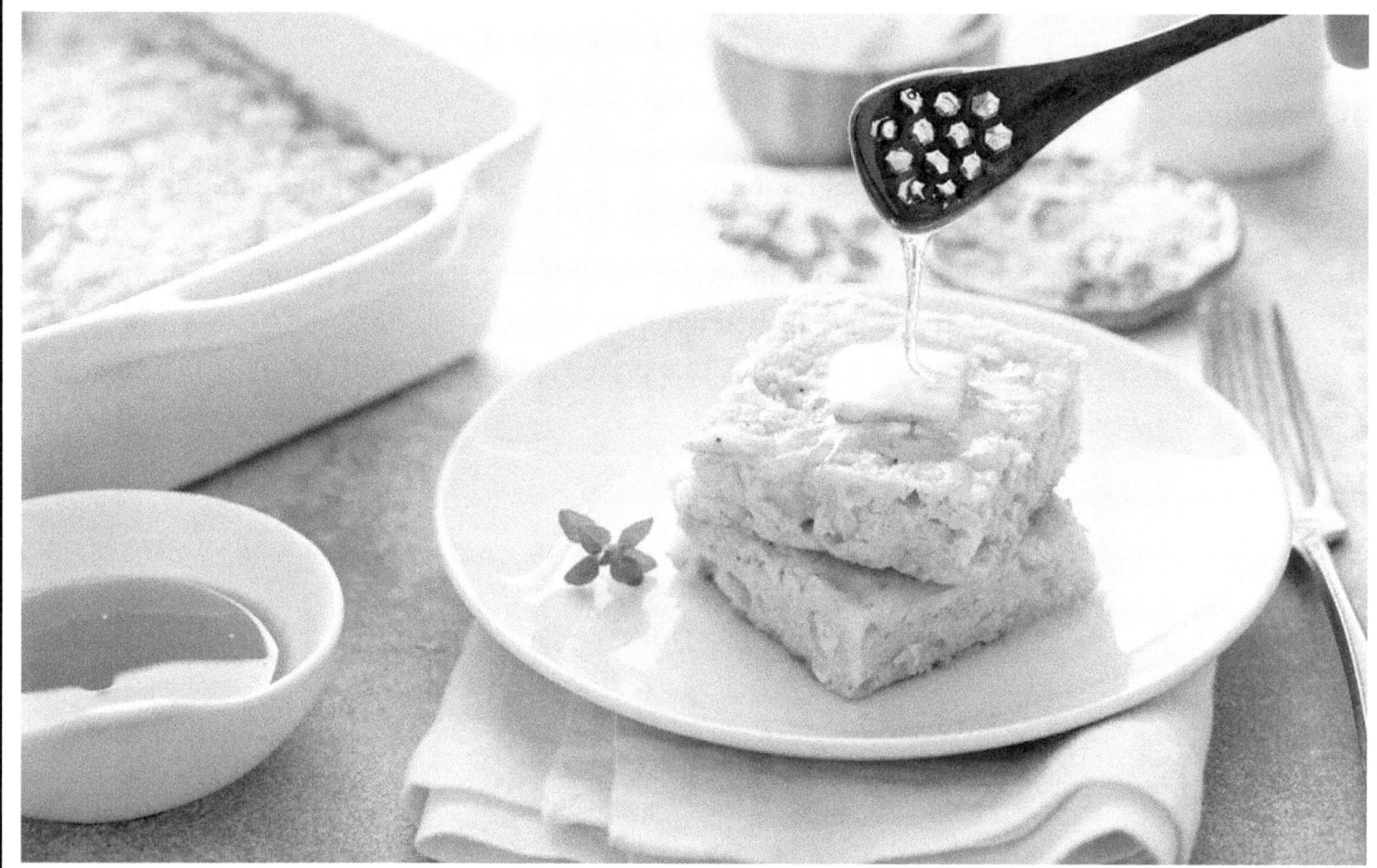

This is the recipe for you if you prefer sweet cornbread. This is a family favorite.

Nutrition

Calories: 189 | Protein: 3.1g | Fat: 7.4g | Cholesterol: 17.1mg | Sodium: 353.9mg

Carbohydrates: 28.2g

Ingredients

- ⅓ cup vegetable oil
- ⅔ Cup white sugar
- 1 cup all-purpose flour
- 1 cup milk
- 1 cup yellow cornmeal
- 1 egg
- 1 teaspoon salt
- 3 ½ teaspoons baking powder

Instructions

1. Preheat the oven to 400 degrees Fahrenheit. A 9-inch round cake pan must be lightly greased or sprayed.
2. Combine flour, cornmeal, sugar, salt, and baking powder in a large mixing basin. Combine the egg, milk, and vegetable oil in a large mixing bowl. Pour the batter into the pan that has been prepared.
3. Bake for twenty to twenty-five minutes in a preheated oven or until a toothpick inserted in the center of the loaf comes out clean.

VEGAN JALAPENO CORNBREAD IN THE AIR FRYER

Preparation: 10 Minutes

Cook: 20 Minutes

Servings: 6

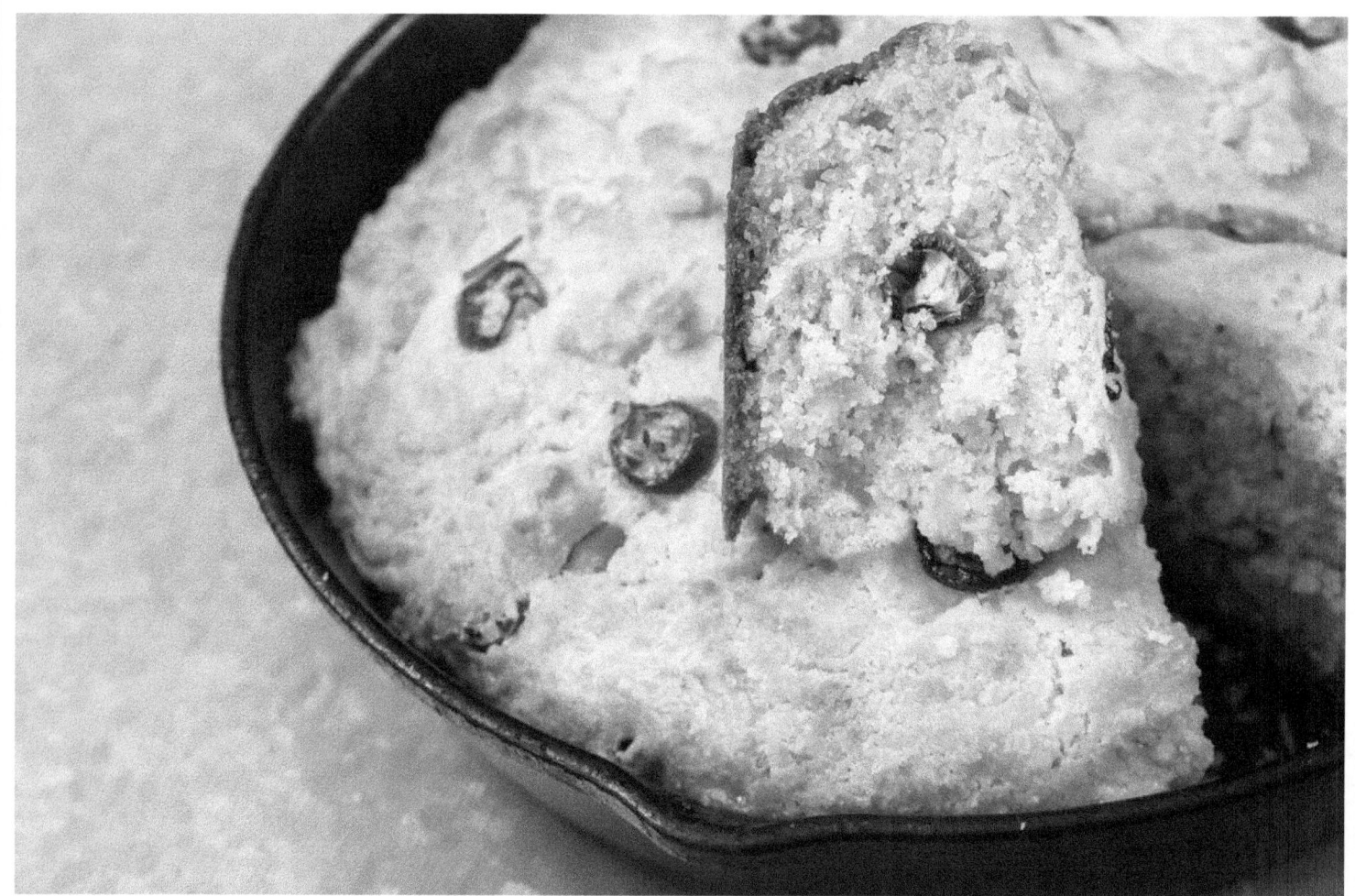

Vegan cornbread that is tasty, spicy, and rich and made in the air fryer! Please keep in mind that the results may vary depending on the brand and size. You'll need an air fryer with a 6-inch inner pot that can be added.

Nutrition

Calories: 294 | Protein: 6.2g | Fat: 13.9g | Sodium: 485.7mg | Carbohydrates: 37g

Ingredients

- ¼ cup nutritional yeast
- ⅓ cup vegetable oil
- ½ teaspoon ground black pepper
- ⅔ cup all-purpose flour
- 1 cup stone-ground yellow cornmeal
- 1 cup unsweetened almond milk
- 1 large jalapeno pepper, seeded and minced, or to taste
- 1 tablespoon flaxseed meal
- 1 teaspoon kosher salt
- 2 tablespoons white sugar
- 2 ¼ teaspoons baking powder
- 3 tablespoons water
- cooking spray

Instructions

1. In a small bowl, combine water and flaxseed meal and set aside for ten minutes.
2. Meanwhile, preheat an air fryer to 350 degrees F as directed by the manufacturer. Cooking spray a 6-inch heat-resistant inner pot
3. In a medium mixing bowl, combine cornmeal, flour, nutritional yeast, sugar, baking powder, salt, and pepper. Stir in the flaxseed and water combination, almond milk, and oil until everything is combined and no lumps remain. Pour into the prepared pot with the jalapeno and place in the air fryer.
4. Cook for fifteen minutes in a preheated air fryer.
5. Remove the inner pot with tongs, flip the cornbread, and continue to air fry for another five minutes or until a toothpick inserted in the center comes out clean. Warm the dish before serving.

ANGIE'S DILLY CASSEROLE BREAD

Preparation: 15 Minutes

Cook: 35 Minutes

Servings: 8

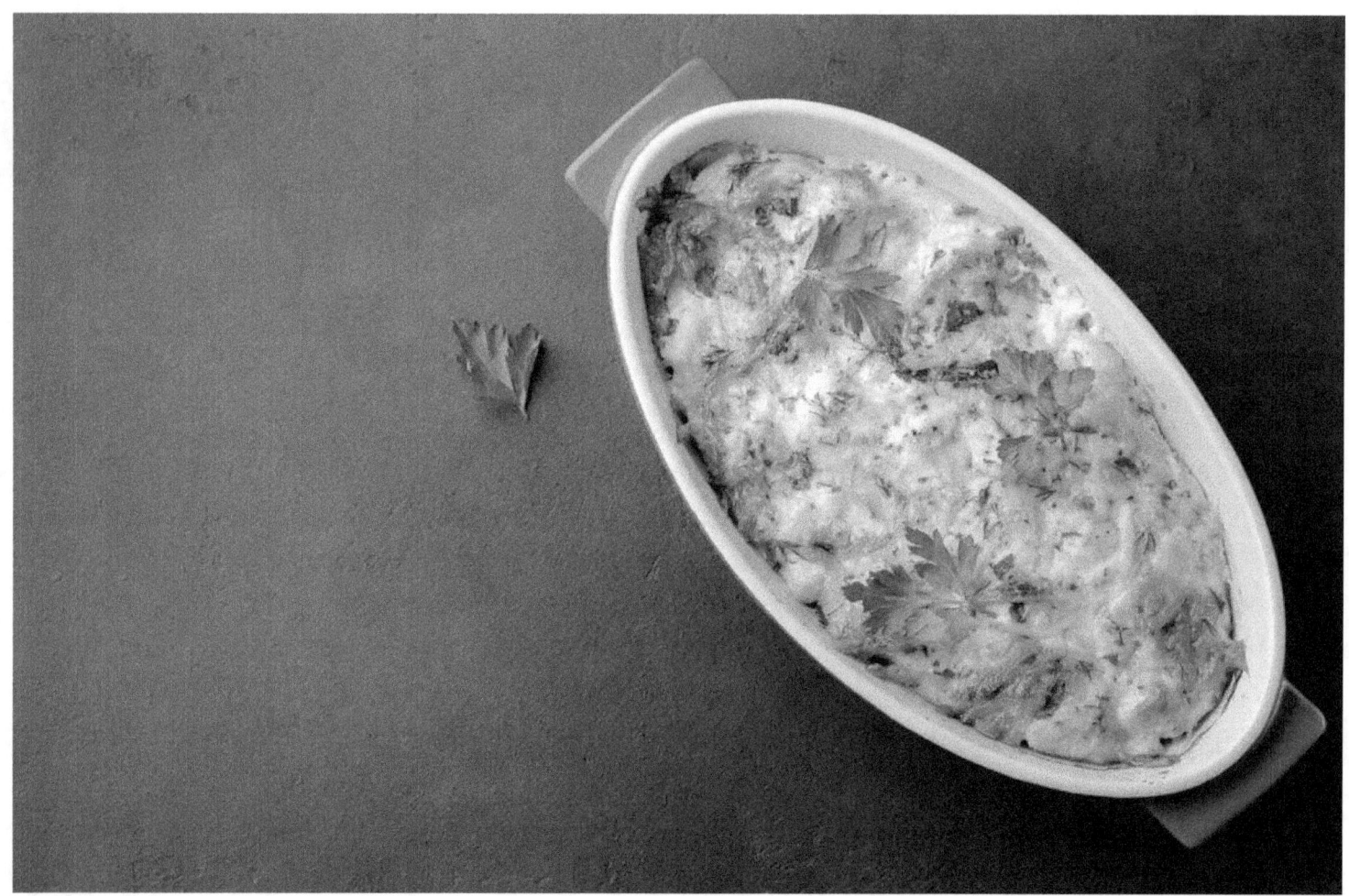

This dense, flavorful bread rises to the top of the oven. It's a recipe passed down through the generations. It's even delicious when it's toasted and slathered in butter

Nutrition

Calories: 196 | Protein: 8.4g | Cholesterol: 31.3mg | Sodium: 483.8mg

Carbohydrates: 31.7g | Fat: 3.8g

Ingredients

- ¼ cup warm water
- ¼ teaspoon baking soda
- 1 package active dry yeast
- 1 cup cottage cheese, room temperature
- 1 egg
- 1 pinch salt
- 1 tablespoon butter, room temperature, plus more as needed
- 1 tablespoon dried minced onion
- 1 teaspoon salt
- 2 tablespoons white sugar
- 2 teaspoons dill seed
- 2 ¼ cups all-purpose flour, or more if needed

Instructions

1. Allow yeast to soften in warm water for ten minutes.
2. In a large mixing bowl, combine cottage cheese, sugar, butter, 1 teaspoon salt, and baking soda. Mix the dill seed, dried onion, egg, and yeast mixture in a mixing bowl. Mix thoroughly. Add the flour in 1/4 cup increments, stirring thoroughly after each addition. If the dough is too sticky, add a tablespoon or two more flour.
3. Cover bowl with a clean cotton kitchen towel and set aside in a warm area for about one hour or until doubled in size.
4. Preheat the oven to 350 degrees Fahrenheit. Butter a 1 1/2 to 2-quart baking dish generously.
5. To release bubbles, gently stir the dough. Transfer to the baking dish that has been prepared. Bake for 35 minutes in a preheated oven until golden brown. Remove from the oven and brush the top with butter before seasoning with a touch of salt. Allow bread to cool for five minutes before transferring to a cooling rack.

ZA'ATAR PULL-APART BREAD ROLLS

Preparation: 20 Minutes

Cook: 25 Minutes

Servings: 12

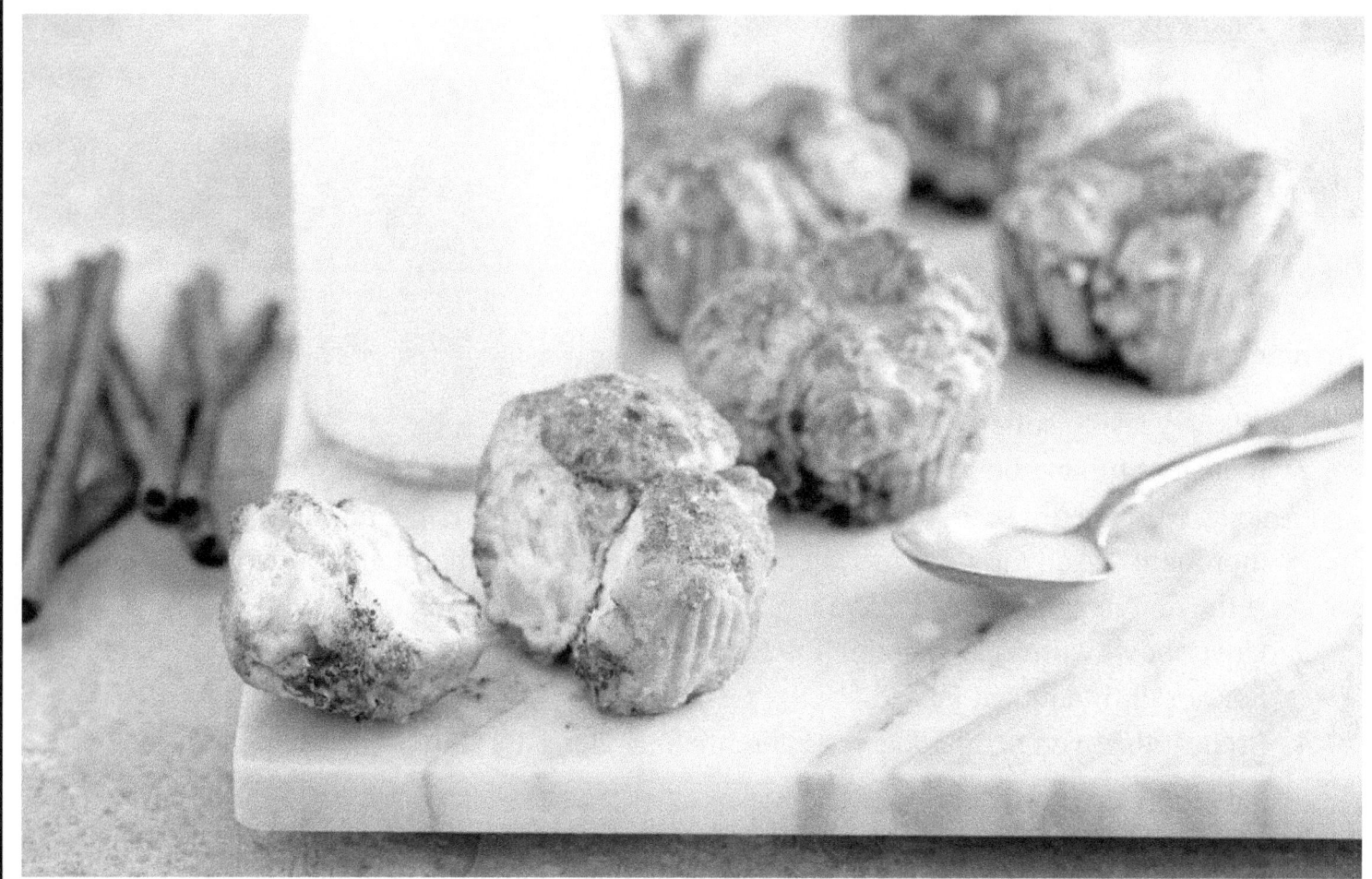

Monkey bread and pull-apart bread don't have to be sweet! This easy handmade dough is coated in za'atar, a tasty Middle Eastern herb mix, and baked in muffin tins. For brunch, serve with labneh, olives, and fresh mint.

Nutrition

Calories: 244 | Protein: 5.5g | Cholesterol: 37.4mg | Sodium: 130.3mg

Carbohydrates: 28.9g | Fat: 12g

Ingredients

- ⅓ cup olive oil
- ½ cup za'atar, divided
- ½ teaspoon fine sea salt
- ⅔ cup warm whole milk
- 1 package active dry yeast
- 1 teaspoon white sugar
- 2 eggs
- 2 tablespoons olive oil
- 2 tablespoons salted butter, melted
- 3 ¼ cups all-purpose flour, divided
- cooking spray

Instructions

1. In the bowl of a stand mixer fitted with the paddle attachment, combine warm milk, yeast, and sugar. Allow five to ten minutes for the mixture to froth up.
2. At low speed, beat the milk mixture. 1 cup flour, beaten until just mixed Combine the melted butter, 2 tablespoons olive oil, and 1/2 cup flour in a mixing bowl. Incorporate the eggs. Combine the remaining 1 3/4 cup flour and the salt in a bowl and mix. In a mixing bowl, combine all of the ingredients and beat until a soft, sticky dough forms.
3. Coat a large mixing bowl with cooking spray and add the dough. Cover loosely and let rise for 1 hour, or until doubled in size.
4. Preheat the oven to 350 degrees Fahrenheit. Using cooking spray, grease a 12-cup muffin tray.
5. Gently press the dough down. Make 36 small dough balls by pinching off 36 small pieces of dough and rolling them into balls.
6. In a mixing dish, combine 6 teaspoons za'atar and 1/3 cup olive oil. In each muffin cup, place three dough balls. Coat all sides of the dough balls with the oil mixture. Sprinkle the remaining 2 tablespoons za'atar over the dough.
7. Grease a muffin tray and cover it loosely with plastic wrap. Allow dough balls to rise for about twenty-five minutes or until they puff out over the tin's rim.
8. Preheat the oven to 350°F and bake until golden and puffy, about twenty-five minutes. In the pan, cool for five minutes. Remove from the pan and let it get cool for another five minutes on a wire rack.

LEBANESE MOUNTAIN BREAD

Preparation: *20 Minutes*

Cook: *Minutes*

Servings: *8*

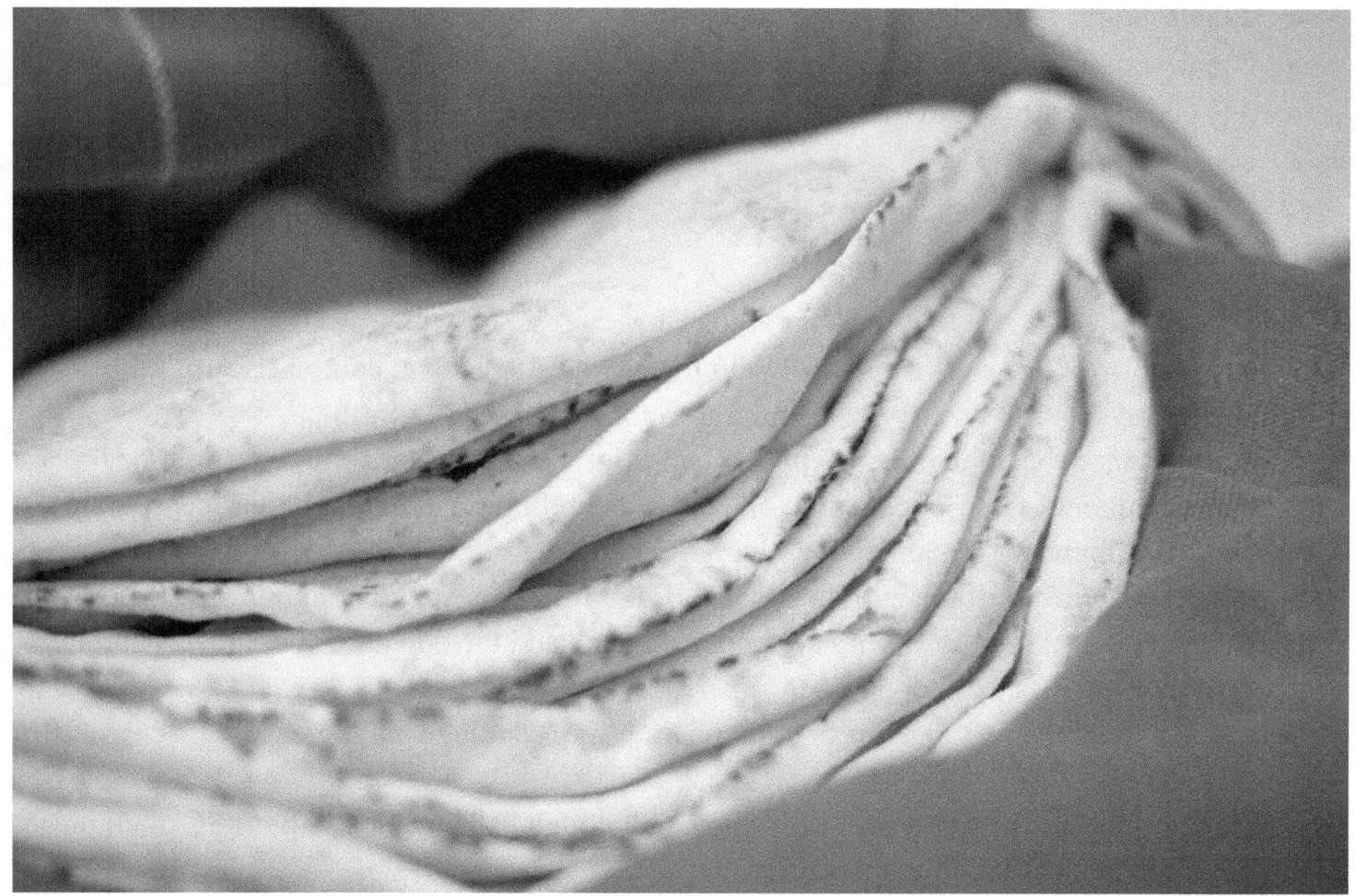

This flatbread reminds me of my early childhood when a Syrian lady baked it. Who lived across the street from my grandmother and always offered us some. The bread has a distinctive texture, a lovely appearance, and a technique that is easy to master.

Nutrition

Calories: 47 | Protein: 1.2g | Fat: 1.9g | Sodium: 180.9mg | Carbohydrates: 6.4g

Ingredients

- ½ cup bread flour
- ½ cup warm water
- ¾ teaspoon kosher salt
- 1 cup bread flour, or more as needed
- 1 tablespoon olive oil, plus extra to coat the bowl
- 1 teaspoon active dry yeast
- 1 teaspoon white sugar

Instructions

1. In a mixing dish, combine 1/2 cup flour, yeast, and sugar. Fill the container halfway with warm water. Whisk together thoroughly, two to three minutes. Cover bowl and set aside for thirty to sixty minutes, or until mixture begins to bubble. Drizzle in the olive oil, then season with salt and 1 cup flour. Mix until the dough forms a sticky dough ball that pulls away from the bowl's sides. If the mixture appears to be excessively wet, add a little more flour.
2. Flour a work surface lightly. Knead the dough for about two minutes, or until it is soft, pliable, and slightly elastic. In a bowl, pour a few drops of olive oil. Turn the dough ball in the bowl to coat the surface with oil.
3. Cover the bowl and keep it in a warm area. Allow the dough to rise for sixty to ninety minutes or until it has doubled in size. Transfer dough to work surface and knead for one minute to remove air bubbles. Refrigerate for eight hours or overnight in a zip-top plastic bag.
4. Dust a work surface lightly with flour; dough can be sticky, so be sure to use enough flour to keep it from adhering to the surface or your hands. Break off a little piece of dough about the size of a golf ball. Make a smooth ball out of the dough. Flatten and roll out into a 1/8-inch thick circle.
5. Invert a smooth mixing bowl onto a work surface and dust the bottom lightly with flour. Stretch the dough lightly before placing it on the floured surface of the inverted bowl. Stretch the dough evenly along the sides of the bowl, working your way around the edges until it is very thin and translucent, or as thin as it will go without tearing.
6. A cast-iron skillet should be heated at high heat. Remove the dough circle from the bottom of the bowl with floured hands. Place in a heated skillet. Cook for forty-five to sixty seconds per side, or until blisters appear and begin to brown. Transfer to a dish and cover, inverting the dish over the bread to enable steam to escape and keep it moist and supple.

MUSTARD WHEAT RYE SANDWICH BREAD

Preparation: 5 Minutes

Cook: 3 Hours

Servings: 12

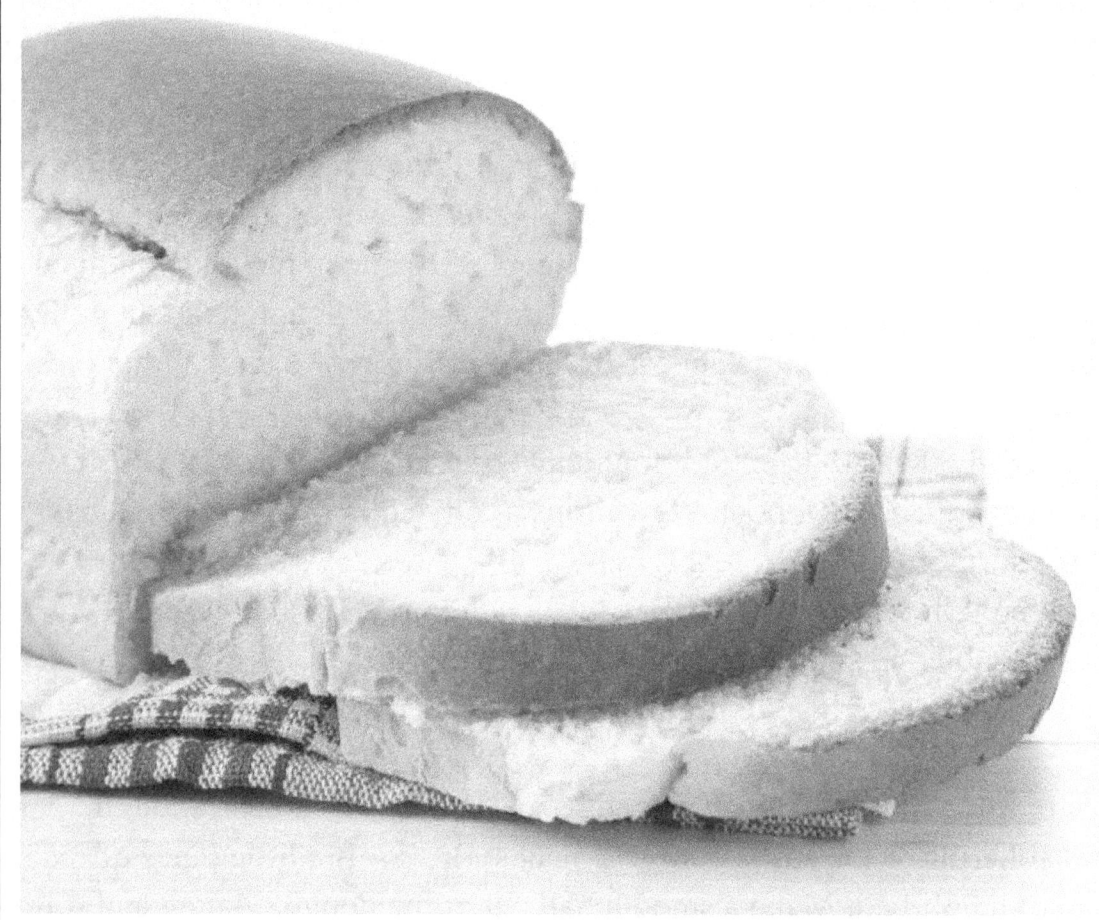

This bread is ideal for sandwiches. It's perfect for a grilled cheese.

Nutrition

Calories: 163 | Protein: 4.5g | Fat: 2.7g | Sodium: 252.3mg | Carbohydrates: 29.9g

Ingredients

- ½ cup Dijon-style prepared mustard
- ⅔ cup rye flour
- ⅔ cup whole wheat flour
- 1 cup warm water
- 1 ½ tablespoons molasses
- 1 ½ tablespoon vital wheat gluten
- 2 cups unbleached all-purpose flour
- 2 tablespoons olive oil
- 2 ½ teaspoons active dry yeast

Instructions

1. Place all of the ingredients in the bread machine pan in the manufacturer's recommended order.
2. Start the machine with the Basic or White Bread preset.

MONKEY BREAD

Preparation: 15 Minutes

Cook: 35 Minutes

Servings: 15

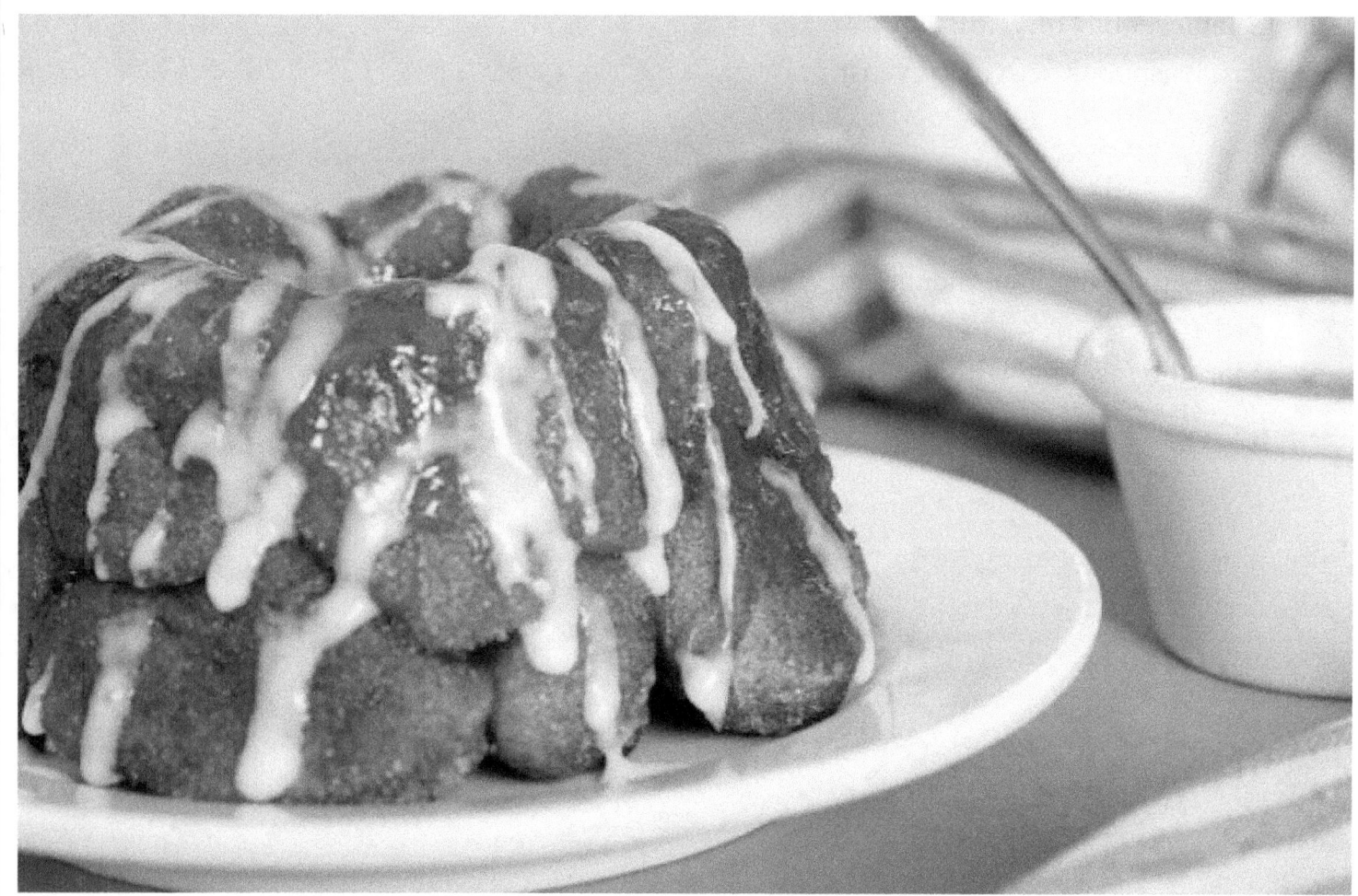

Biscuits with cinnamon that have been refrigerated bake in a tube pan. Leah, my seven-year-old daughter, adores her Monkey Bread. Enjoy

Nutrition

Calories: 418 | Protein: 5.3g | Cholesterol: 0.7mg | Sodium: 746.2mg

Carbohydrates: 61.5g | Fat: 17.7g

Ingredients

- ½ cup margarine
- ½ cup raisins
- 1 cup packed brown sugar
- 1 cup white sugar
- 2 teaspoons ground cinnamon
- 3 packages refrigerated biscuit dough
- ½ cup chopped walnuts (optional)

Instructions

1. Preheat oven to 350 degrees F. Grease one 9 or 10-inch tube
2. In a plastic bag, combine white sugar and cinnamon. Make quarters out of the biscuits. Shake 6 to 8 biscuit pieces in the sugar-cinnamon mix. Place the pieces in the prepared pan's bottom. Continue coating and placing biscuits in the pan until all biscuits are coated. If you're using nuts and raisins, sprinkle them on top of the biscuits as you go.
3. Melt the margarine and brown sugar in a small saucepan over medium heat. After one minute at a boil, Pour the mixture over the biscuits.
4. Preheat oven to 350 and bake for thirty-five minutes. Allow ten minutes for the bread to cool in the pan before turning it out onto a plate. Please don't cut! The bread simply separates.

WHOLE WHEAT HONEY BREAD

Preparation: 5 Minutes

Cook: 3 Hours

Servings: 12

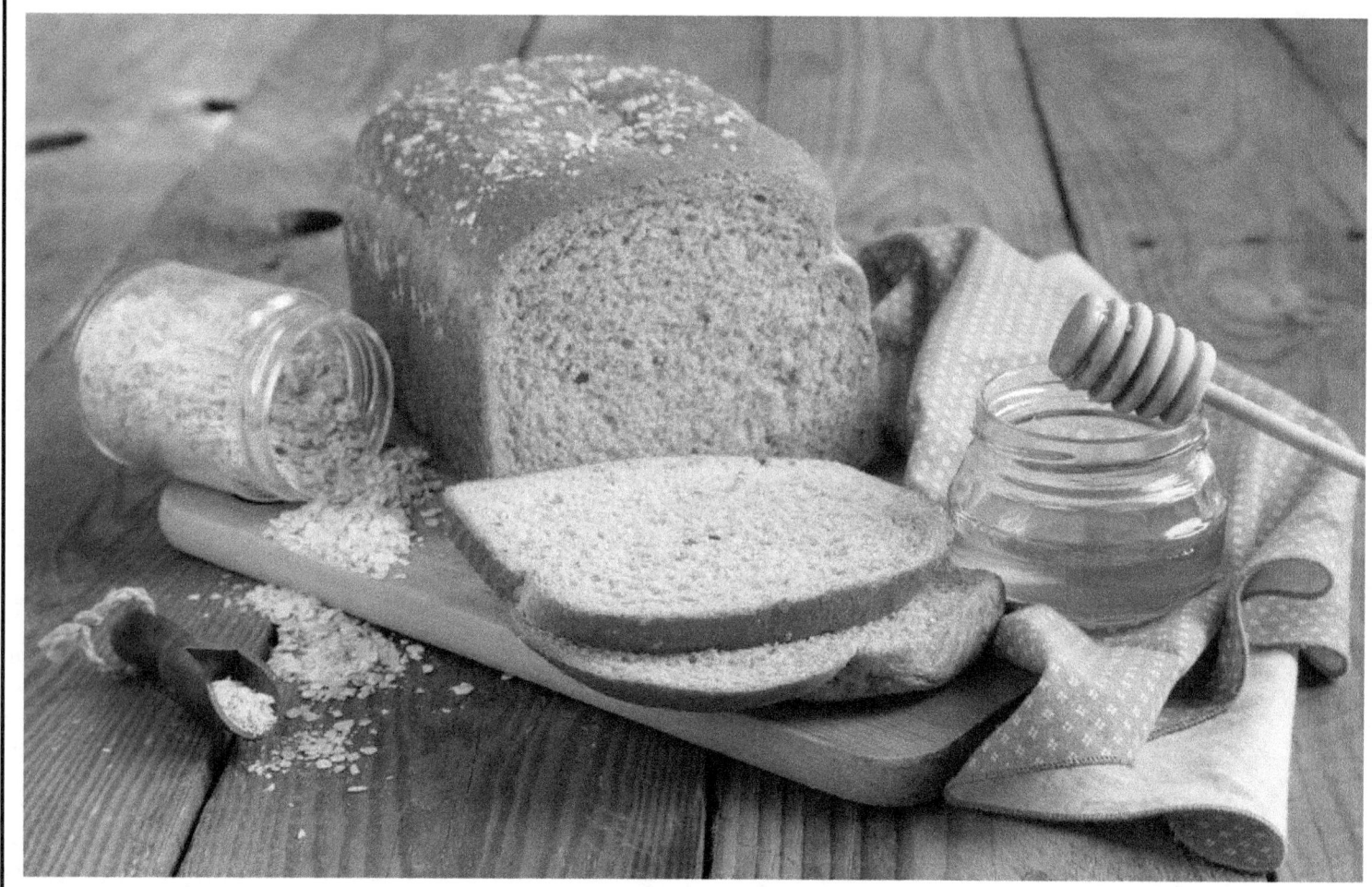

This is a family favorite! Very nice and moist.

Nutrition

Calories: 148 | Protein: 4.6g | Cholesterol: 0.1mg | Sodium: 296.8mg

Carbohydrates: 30g | Fat: 2.2g

Ingredients

- ⅓ cup honey
- 1 tablespoon dry milk powder
- 1 ⅛ cups water
- 1 ½ tablespoons shortening
- 1 ½ teaspoon active dry yeast
- 1 ½ teaspoons salt
- 3 cups whole wheat flour

Instructions

1. Place the ingredients in the bread machine pan in the manufacturer's recommended order.
2. Select the Whole Wheat option, then push the Start button.

LIGHT WHEAT BREAD ROLLS

Preparation: 5 Minutes

Cook: 3 Hours

Servings: 12

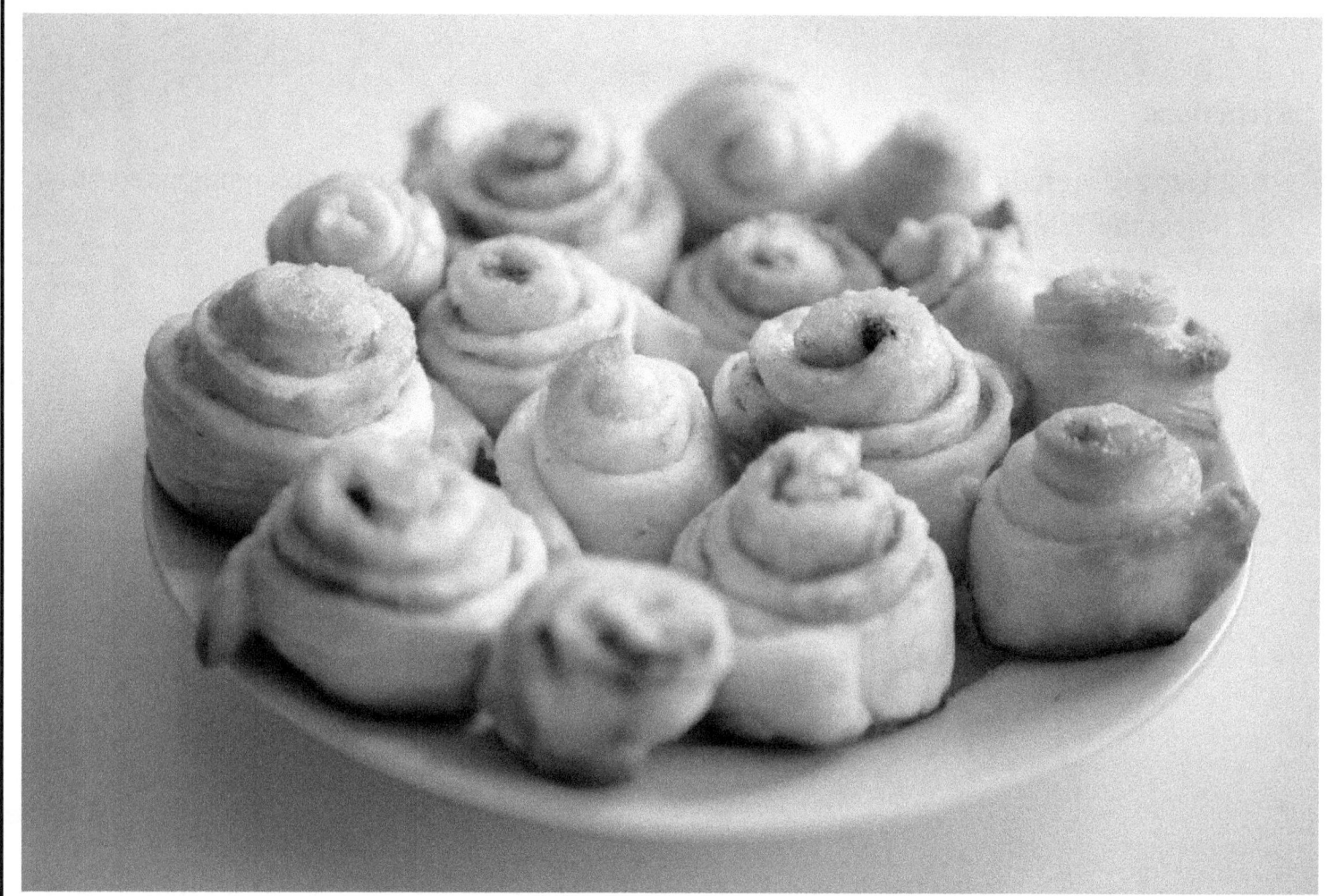

This is a delicious recipe for a light wheat roll that we keep in this recipes book. They're not difficult to make, but they do take a long time to rise.

Nutrition

Calories: 140 | Protein: 3.4g | Cholesterol: 17.9mg | Sodium: 128.7mg

Carbohydrates: 22.5g | Fat: 4.4g

Ingredients

- ¼ cup butter, melted
- ¼ cup butter, melted and cooled
- ½ cup white sugar
- 1 egg, beaten
- 1 teaspoon salt
- 1 ¾ cups warm water
- 2 packages of active dry yeast
- 2 ¼ cups whole wheat flour
- 2 ½ cups all-purpose flour

Instructions

1. Dissolve yeast in warm water in a large mixing dish. Allow ten minutes for the mixture to become creamy.
2. In a large mixing bowl, combine the yeast, sugar, salt, 1/4 cup melted butter, egg, and whole wheat flour. 1/2 cup at a time, stir in all-purpose flour until dough pulls away from the sides of the dish. Knead the dough on a well-floured surface for about eight minutes, or until smooth and elastic. Lightly oil a large mixing bowl, then add the dough and toss to coat.
3. Cover with a moist towel and set aside in a warm place to rise for one hour or until doubled in volume.
4. Allow dough to rise in a warm area until it has doubled in size, about thirty minutes.
5. Grease 2 dozen muffin cups. Divide dough into two equal parts after punching it down. Each one will be rolled into a 6x14-inch rectangle and cut into twelve 7x1-inch strips. Spiralize the strips and set them in muffin cups. Using melted butter, brush the tops of the cookies. Allow to rise for forty minutes, or until doubled in mass, uncovered in a warm location.
6. Preheat oven to 400 degrees F. Bake for twelve to fifteen minutes, or until golden brown. Remove from oven, and brush again with melted butter.

FLAX AND SUNFLOWER SEED BREAD

Preparation: 10 Minutes

Cook: 30 min

Servings: 15

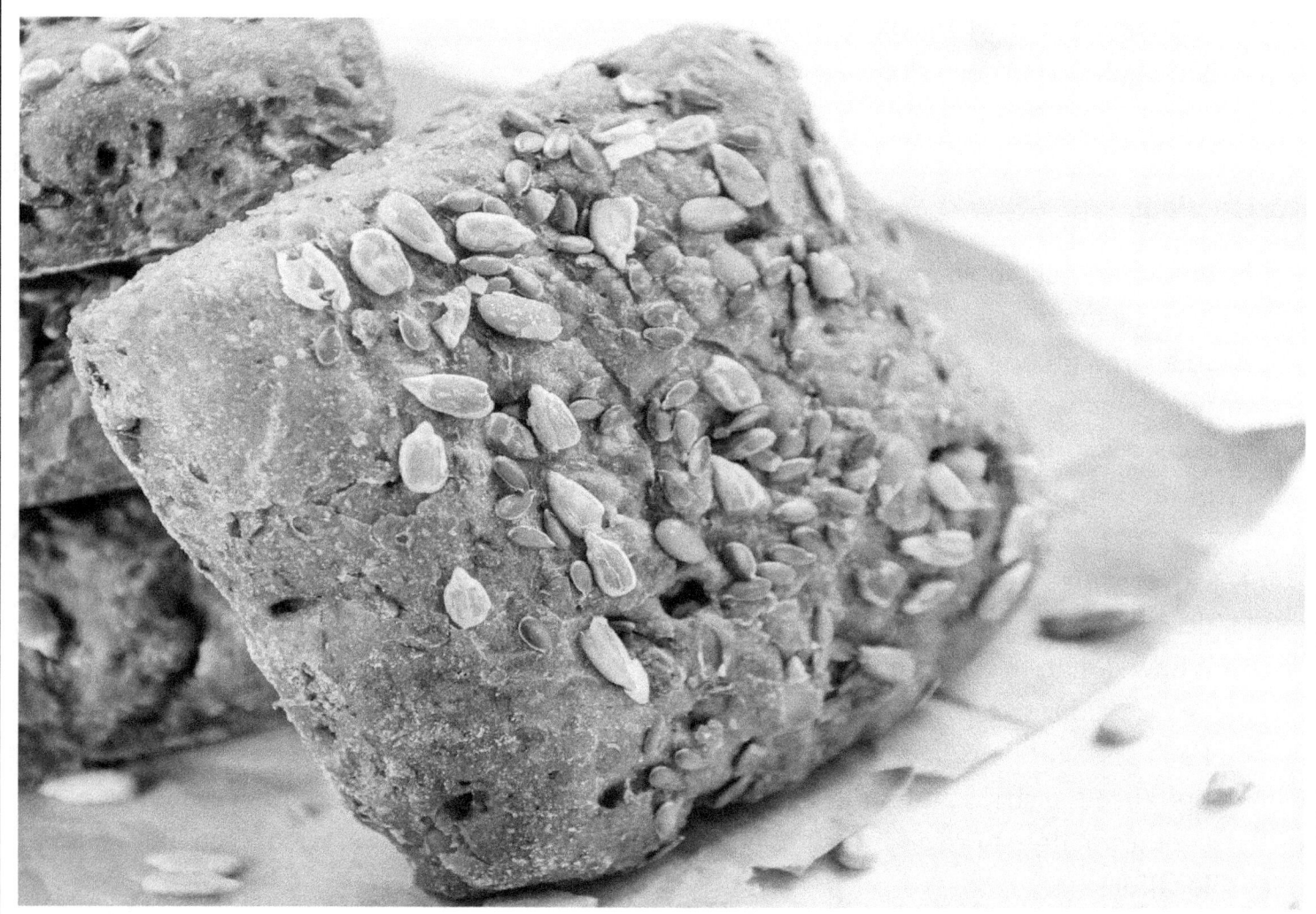

This is a delicious bread for seed lovers and one of the best in the book.

Nutrition

Calories: 140 | Protein: 4.2g | Cholesterol: 4.1mg | Sodium: 168.6mg

Carbohydrates: 22.7g | Fat: 4.2g

Ingredients

- ½ cup flax seeds
- ½ cup sunflower seeds
- 1 teaspoon active dry yeast
- 1 teaspoon salt
- 1 ⅓ cups water
- 1 ⅓ cups whole wheat bread flour
- 1 ½ cups bread flour
- 2 tablespoons butter, softened
- 3 tablespoons honey

Instructions

1. In the bread machine pan, place all ingredients in the order indicated by the manufacturer.
2. Select the Basic White Cycle and press the Start button. When the Knead Cycle's signal sounds, add the sunflower seeds.

DEE'S HEALTH BREAD

Preparation: 10 Minutes

Cook: 30 min

Servings: 72

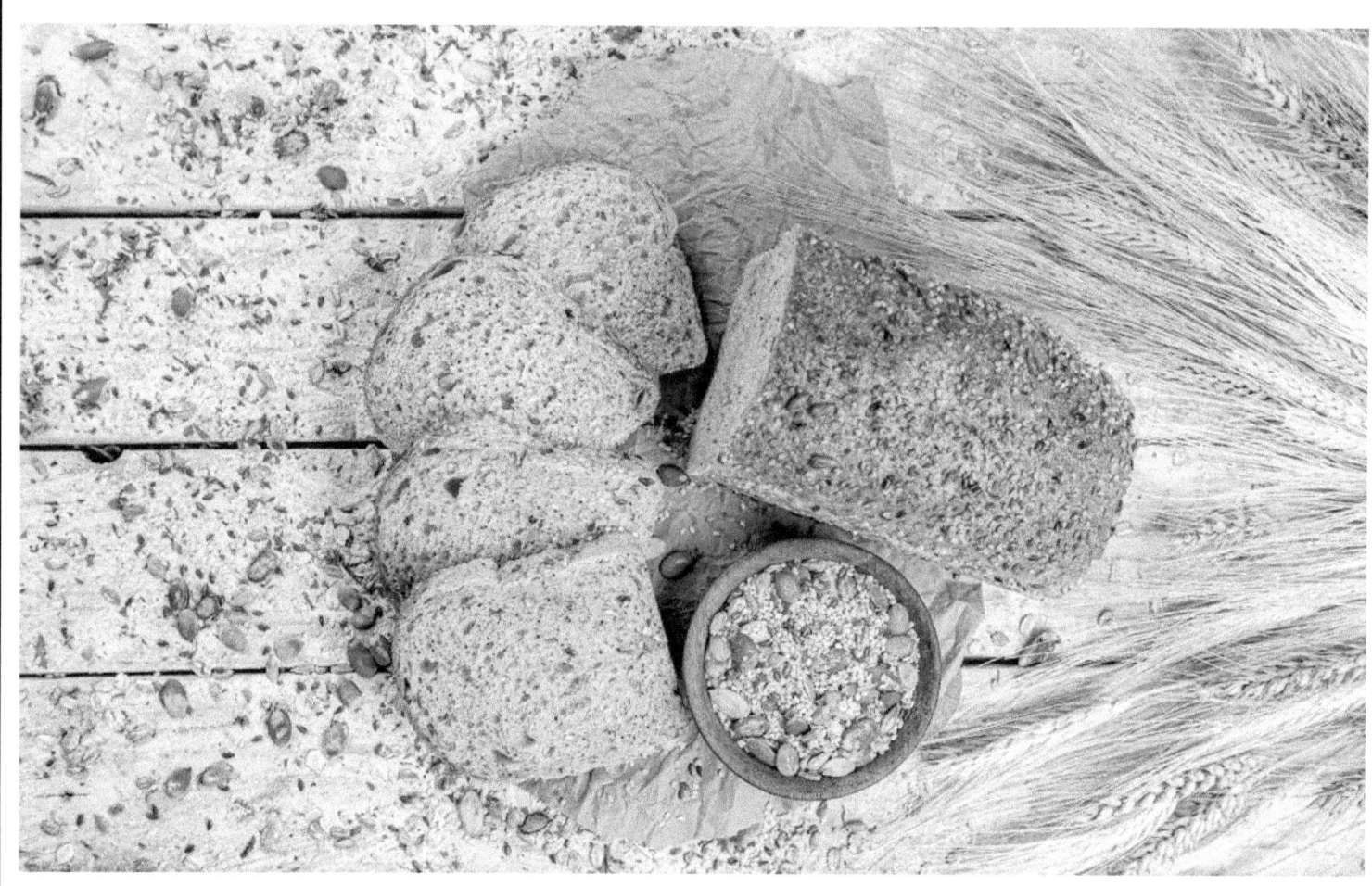

Sunflower seeds, cracked wheat, and honey on whole-wheat bread.

Nutrition

Calories: 94 | Protein: 3g | Cholesterol: 5.2mg | Sodium: 132.5mg

Carbohydrates: 16.6g | Fat: 2.2g

Ingredients

- ¼ cup cracked wheat
- ¼ cup flax seed
- ¼ cup honey
- ¼ cup molasses
- ¼ cup sunflower seeds
- ½ cup vegetable oil
- ½ cup warm water
- 1 teaspoon white sugar
- 2 eggs
- 2 tablespoons active dry yeast
- 2 tablespoons lemon juice
- 3 ½ cups warm water
- 4 cups bread flour
- 4 teaspoons salt
- 7 cups whole wheat flour

Instructions

1. Dissolve the yeast and sugar in 1/2 cup warm water in a small bowl. Combine the remaining 3 1/2 cups warm water, honey, molasses, oil, eggs, and lemon juice in a large mixing bowl. Mix thoroughly. Stir in the yeast mixture.
2. Add 5 cups whole wheat flour, gradually beating well after each addition. Stir in the flax, cracked wheat, and sunflower seeds.
3. Allow for a twenty-five minutes rest period, or until the mixture is very light. Stir in the salt and the remaining flours until the dough pulls away from the bowl's sides.
4. Knead the dough for ten to fifteen minutes, or until it is smooth and elastic. Place in a greased bowl, cover, and let rise in a warm oven until doubled, about 1 hour.
5. Punch down the dough and roll it into six round balls. Allow for a twenty minutes rest period after covering.
6. Form into loaves and bake until doubled in size, covered. Bake for twenty-five to thirty-five minutes at 375 degrees F.

SEVEN GRAIN BREAD

Preparation: 10 Minutes

Cook: 1 Hour 30 Minutes

Servings: 8

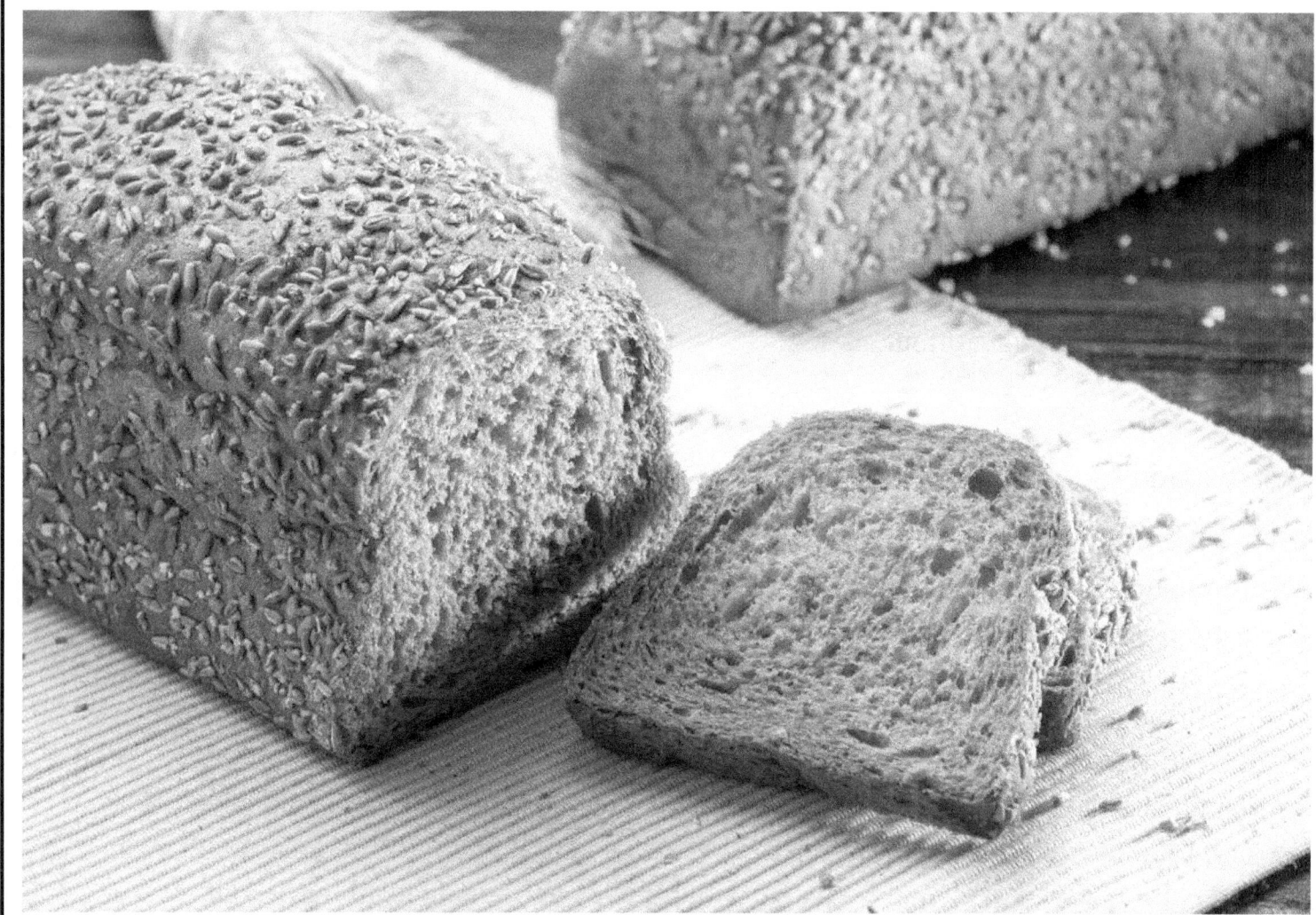

This is wonderful and nutritious bread. It's the 7-grain cereal in the supermarket's bulk area.

Nutrition

Calories: 285 | Protein: 9.8g | Fat: 5.2g | Cholesterol: 23.8mg | Sodium: 629.4mg

Carbohydrates: 50.6g

Ingredients

- ¾ cup 7-grain cereal
- 1 cup whole wheat flour
- 1 egg
- 1 tablespoon active dry yeast
- 1 ⅓ cups warm water
- 2 tablespoons honey
- 2 tablespoons vegetable oil
- 2 teaspoons salt
- 2 ½ cups bread flour
- 3 tablespoons dry milk powder

Instructions

1. Place the ingredients in the bread machine pan in the manufacturer's recommended order.
2. Select the Whole Wheat Bread cycle and press the Start button.

CRACKED WHEAT SOURDOUGH BREAD

Preparation: 10 Minutes

Cook: 1 Hour 30 Minutes

Servings: 24

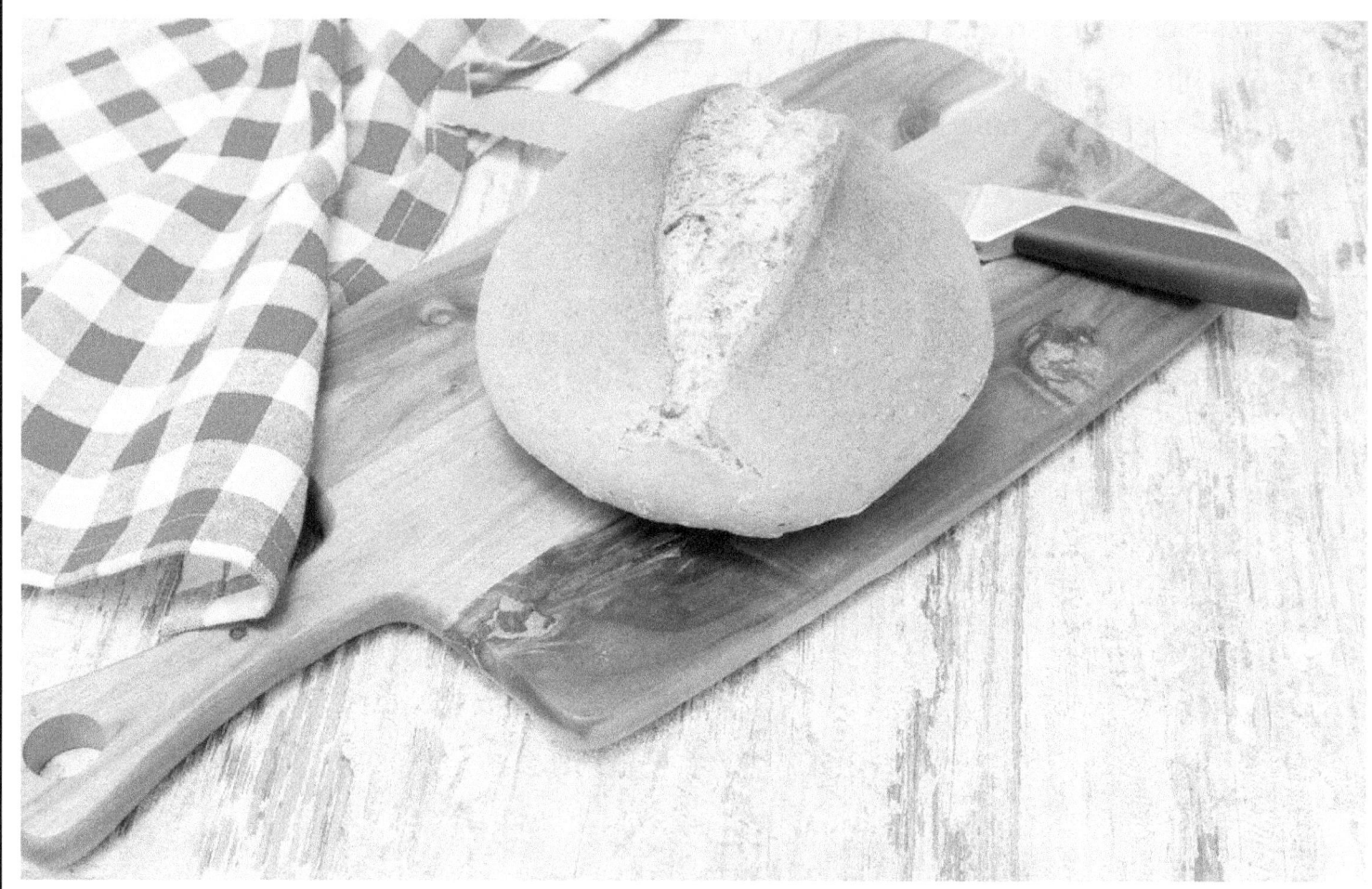

Substantial sourdough bread with grains and seeds. This bread can be made with any decent sourdough starter. The Rye Starter is an example of a starter that can be used.

Nutrition

Calories: 200 | Protein: 7.4g | Cholesterol: 8.1mg | Sodium: 35.8mg

Carbohydrates: 36.1g | Fat: 3.9g

Ingredients

- ¼ cup margarine, melted
- ½ cup flax seed
- ½ cup raw sunflower seeds
- ¾ cup cracked wheat
- ¾ cup nonfat milk
- 1 cup hot water
- 1 egg, beaten
- 2 cups whole wheat flour
- 2 tablespoons honey
- 2 tablespoons molasses
- 2 ½ cups sourdough starter
- 3 ½ cups bread flour

Instructions

1. Crack the wheat in a medium bowl and pour hot water over it. Mix together the melted margarine, molasses, honey, nonfat milk, flaxseed, and sunflower seeds. Allow it to cool lukewarm before adding the sourdough starter.
2. Begin stirring in the flours, one cup at a time, with a large wooden spoon, beginning with the whole wheat flour and ending with the bread flour. When the dough is stiff enough to work with, turn it out onto a floured surface and knead for ten to twelve minutes, using as little flour as possible.
3. When the dough is smooth and elastic, roll it into a ball and place it in a greased bowl, rotating it to coat both sides. Cover and set aside in a warm, draft-free location, and let rise until doubled in volume, approximately one and half hours. Punch down risen dough and leave aside to rise until doubled in bulk, about one hour.
4. Punch down the dough and divide it into two loaves after the second rise is complete. Place dough in two 9x5-inch loaf pans, cover, and let rise until doubled in mass, or until the dough reaches the tops of the pans, about one hour. Brush the tops with an egg wash produced by whisking one whole egg with one tablespoon water until thoroughly combined.
5. Bake for thirty minutes in a preheated 375°F oven; after fifteen minutes, rotate pans and spray with cold water; continue baking until the loaves make a hollow sound when tapped on the top and bottom. Cool for 1ten minutes in the pans on racks before turning out onto racks to cool fully.

WHOLE WHEAT SEED BREAD

Preparation: 20 Minutes

Cook: 40 Minutes

Servings: 48

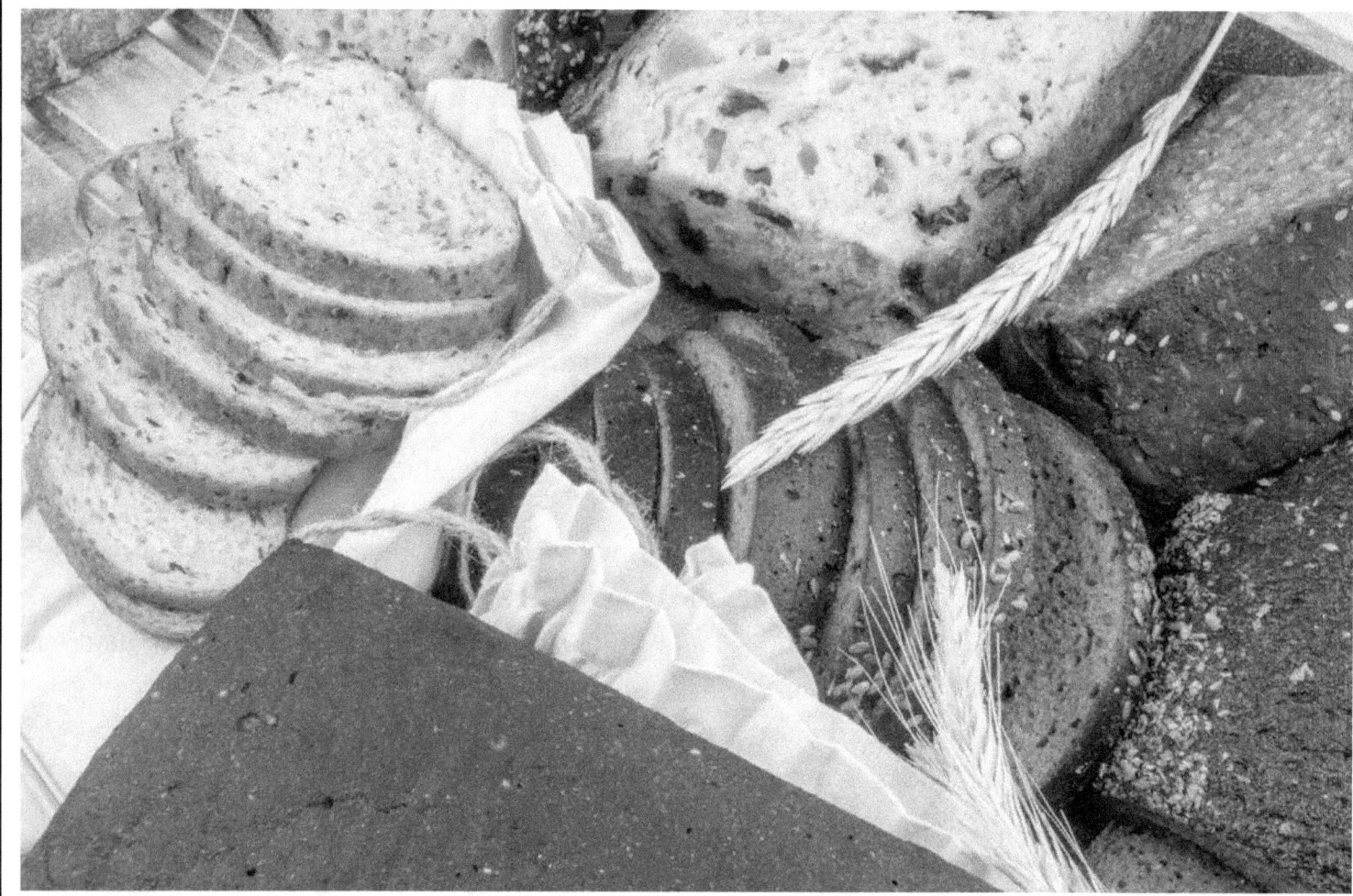

A delightful whole wheat seed bread with honey for sweetness and various seeds for texture and flavor. This is a fantastic everyday bread

Nutrition

Calories: 145 | Protein: 4.4g | Cholesterol: 7.8mg | Sodium: 116.5mg

Carbohydrates: 25.3g | Fat: 3.8g

Ingredients

- ⅓ cup unsweetened applesauce
- ½ cup ground flax seed
- ½ cup honey
- ½ cup molasses
- ½ cup sunflower seeds
- ½ cup vegetable oil
- ½ cup warm water
- ¾ cup cracked wheat
- 1 cup quick-cooking oats
- 1 tablespoon sea salt
- 2 eggs, beaten
- 3 tablespoons active dry yeast
- 3 tablespoons lemon juice
- 3 ½ cups warm water
- 9 cups sifted whole wheat flour

Instructions

1. In a small bowl, whisk 1/2 cup water and applesauce. Dissolve the yeast in the mixture and set aside for five minutes or until creamy. Blend the yeast mixture, 3 1/2 cups warm water, honey, molasses, vegetable oil, lemon juice, and eggs in a large mixing container and stir well to combine.
2. Combine the whole wheat flour, flaxseed, sunflower seeds, cracked wheat, and salt in a separate bowl. Combine the flour, salt, and yeast in a mixing bowl and stir until a smooth dough form. Knead for ten minutes on a lightly floured surface until smooth and elastic. Area in a lightly oiled bowl and cover; let rise until doubled in volume, about one hour in a warm place.
3. Grease four 9x5-inch loaf pans lightly. Punch down the dough and form it into loaves before placing it in the pans. Allow 1 hour for the dough to rise in the pans until it has doubled in bulk.
4. Preheat the oven to 375 degrees Fahrenheit.
5. Bake for forty to fifty minutes, or until the loaves sound hollow when tapped on the bottom when taken from the pan.

SIMPLE WHOLE WHEAT BREAD

Preparation: 20 Minutes

Cook: 40 Minutes

Servings: 48

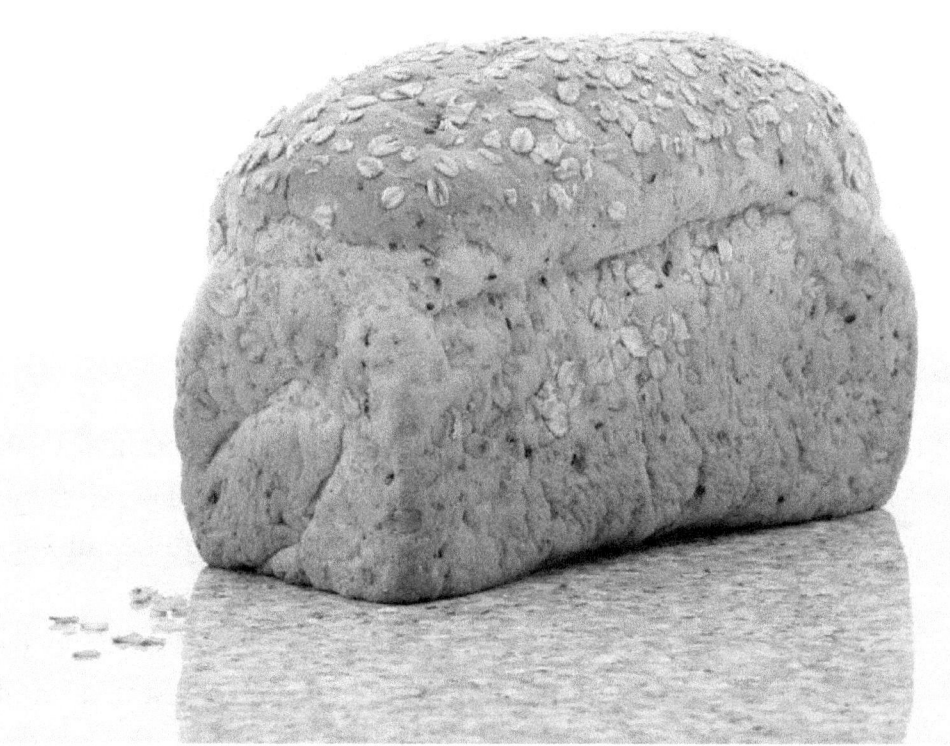

Simply put, this whole wheat bread is delicious and simple to make.

Nutrition

Calories: 145 | Protein: 4.4g | Cholesterol: 7.8mg | Sodium: 116.5mg

Carbohydrates: 25.3g | Fat: 3.8g

Ingredients

- ⅓ cup honey
- ⅓ cup honey
- 1 tablespoon salt
- 2 packages of active dry yeast
- 2 tablespoons butter, melted
- 3 cups warm water
- 3 tablespoons butter, melted
- 3 ½ cups whole wheat flour
- 5 cups bread flour

Instructions

1. Warm water, yeast, and 1/3 cup honey are combined in a large mixing dish. Stir in 5 cups white bread flour until well combined. Set aside for thirty minutes, or until the mixture is large and bubbling.
2. Mix in 3 tablespoons melted butter, 1/3 cup honey, and salt. Stir in 2 cups whole wheat flour. Flour a level surface and knead with whole wheat flour until the dough is no longer sticky but remains sticky to the touch. A total of 2 to 4 cups of whole wheat flour may be required. Place in an oiled dish and turn once to coat the dough's surface. Using a dishtowel, cover the dish.
3. Allow rising until twice in size in a warm location.
4. Punch down the dough and divide it into three loaves. Allow rising in oiled 9 x 5-inch loaf pans until the dough has risen one inch above the pans.
5. Bake for twenty-five to thirty minutes at 350 degrees F; do not overbake. When the loaves are done, lightly spray the tops with 2 tablespoons melted butter or margarine to prevent the crust from hardening. Allow it to cool completely.

SAN FRANCISCO SOURDOUGH BREAD

Preparation: 30 Minutes

Cook: 40 Minutes

Servings: 24

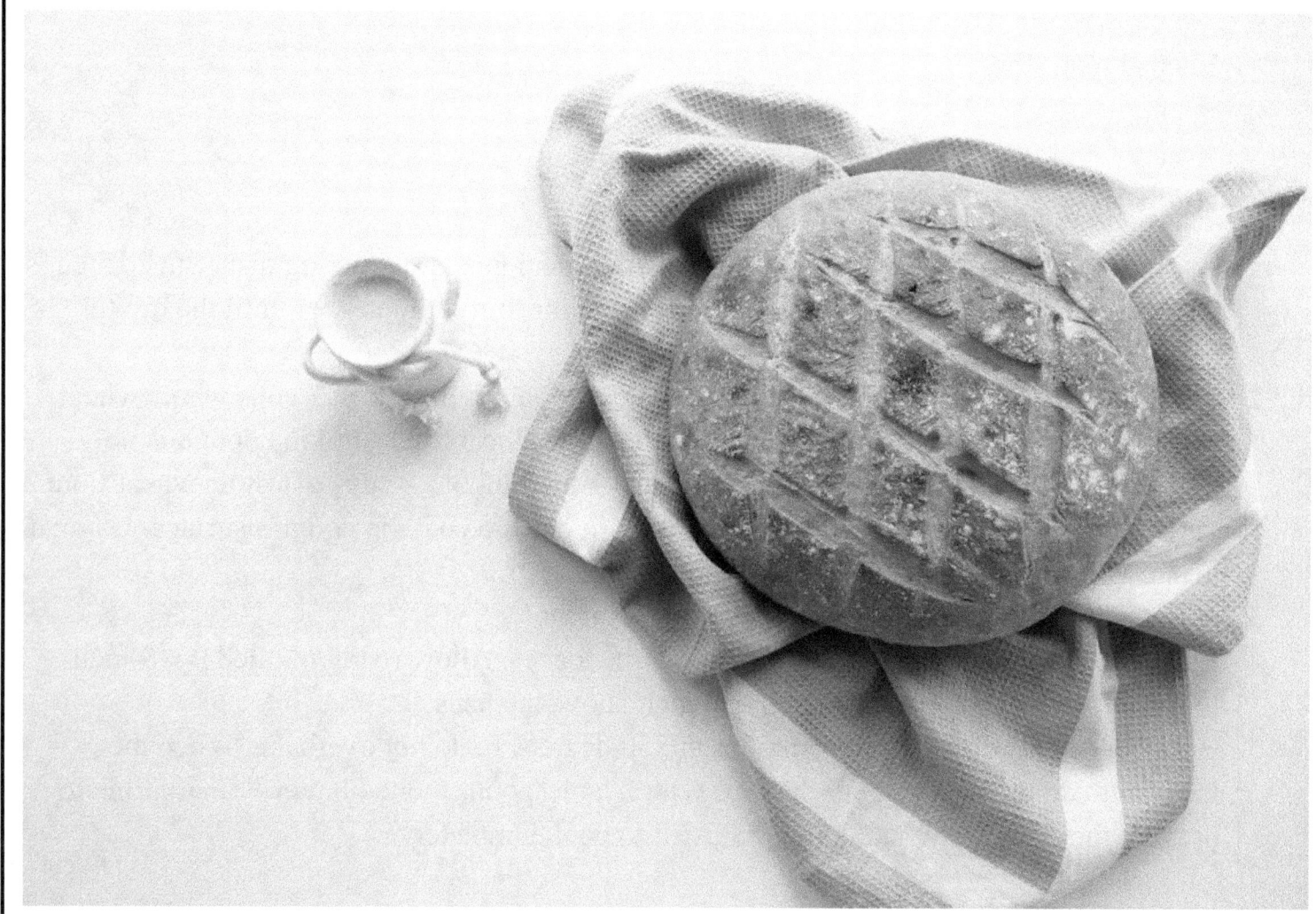

For the finest flavor, use a nice sourdough starter that you've nurtured.

Nutrition

Calories:145 | Protein: 5.1g | Cholesterol: 11.2mg | Sodium: 266.6mg

Carbohydrates: 26.4g | Fat: 2g

Ingredients

- ¼ cup chopped onion
- 1 package active dry yeast
- 1 cup warm milk
- 1 extra-large egg
- 1 tablespoon water
- 1 ½ cups sourdough starter
- 2 tablespoons margarine, softened
- 2 ½ teaspoons salt
- 3 tablespoons white sugar
- 4 ¾ cups bread flour

Instructions

1. Combine 1 cup flour, sugar, salt, and dry yeast in a large mixing bowl. Mix the milk and softened butter or margarine in a mixing bowl. Add the starter and mix well. Gradually add up to 3 3/4 cups flour; depending on your environment, you may need more.
2. Knead the dough for around eight to ten minutes on a floured surface. Place in an oiled mixing bowl, turn once to coat with oil, and cover. Allow for an hour of rising time or until the volume has doubled.
3. Allow fifteen minutes to recover after punching down. Form loaves with the dough. Place on a baking sheet that has been buttered. Allow for an hour of rising time or until the dough has doubled in size.
4. Brush the tops of the loaves with egg wash and sprinkle with chopped onion.
5. Bake for thirty minutes at 375 degrees F until done.

PLAIN AND SIMPLE SOURDOUGH BREAD

Preparation: 5 Minutes

Cook: 3 Hours

Servings: 12

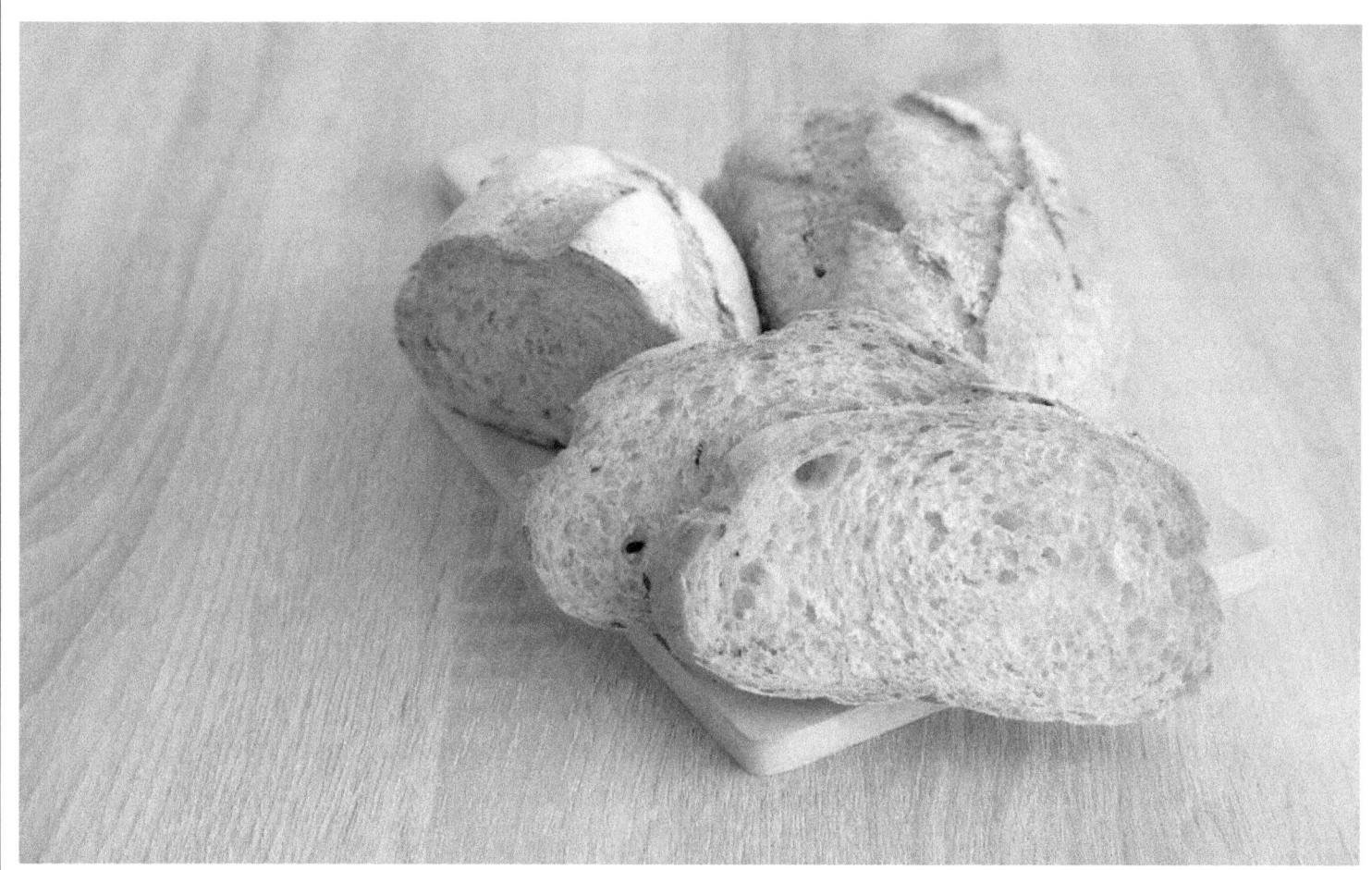

For the bread machine, a simple sourdough bread.

Nutrition

Calories: 31 | Protein: 1.6g | Cholesterol: 0.1mg | Sodium: 295.7mg

Carbohydrates: 6g | Fat: 0.1g

Ingredients

- ¾ cup warm water
- 1 cup sourdough starter
- 1 ½ teaspoon active dry yeast
- 1 ½ teaspoons salt
- 2 ⅔ cups bread flour

Instructions

1. All ingredients must be added in the sequence recommended by your manufacturer.
2. Select the white bread option and press the start button.

FRENCH COUNTRY BREAD

Preparation: 30 Minutes

Cook: 40 Minutes

Servings: 30

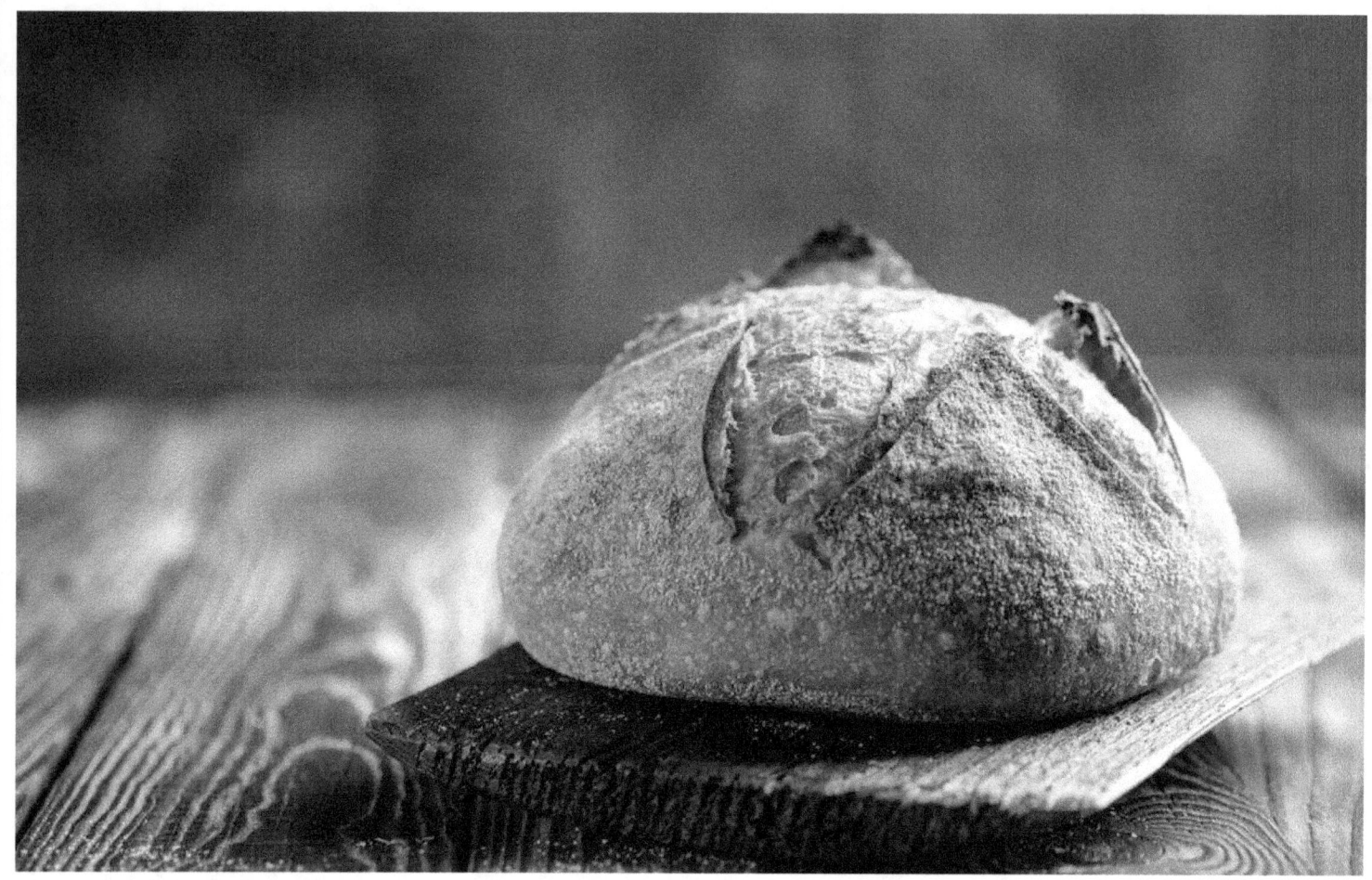

A plain country bread in the European manner. There's just enough whole wheat to give it some flavor without making it too heavy.

Nutrition

Calories: 101 | Protein: 3.6g | Fat: 0.5g | Sodium: 156.6mg | Carbohydrates: 20.4g

Ingredients

- ½ teaspoon active dry yeast
- 1 cup warm water
- 1 cup whole wheat flour
- 1 ½ cups bread flour
- 2 cups warm water
- 2 teaspoons active dry yeast
- 2 teaspoons salt
- 4 ½ cups bread flour, divided

Instructions

1. This starter will be made the night before baking the bread: 1/2 teaspoon active dry yeast, dissolved in 1 cup warm water in a medium non-metal mixing bowl Mix in 1 1/2 cup bread flour thoroughly. Allow sitting at room temperature overnight.
2. The next day, dissolve the 2 teaspoons yeast in 2 cups warm water in a large mixing dish. Stir in the starter, whole wheat flour, 3 cups bread flour, and salt until everything is thoroughly incorporated. Add 1/2 cup at a time, then add remaining bread flour, mixing well after each addition.
3. Lightly grease a large mixing bowl, then set the dough in it and turn to coat it in oil. Cover with a moist towel and set aside in a warm place to rise for one hour or until doubled in volume.
4. Grease two 9x5-inch loaf pans. Turn the dough out onto a lightly floured surface to deflate it. Form the dough into two loaves by dividing it into two equal portions. Place the loaves in the pans that have been prepared. Allow forty-five minutes for the loaves to rise after being covered with a moist cloth. Preheat oven to 425 degrees Fahrenheit.
5. Bake for thirty minutes in a preheated oven or until the top is golden brown and the bottom sounds hollow when tapped.

NO-KNEAD ARTISAN STYLE BREAD

Preparation: 2 Hours 15 Minutes

Cook: 45 Minutes

Servings: 6

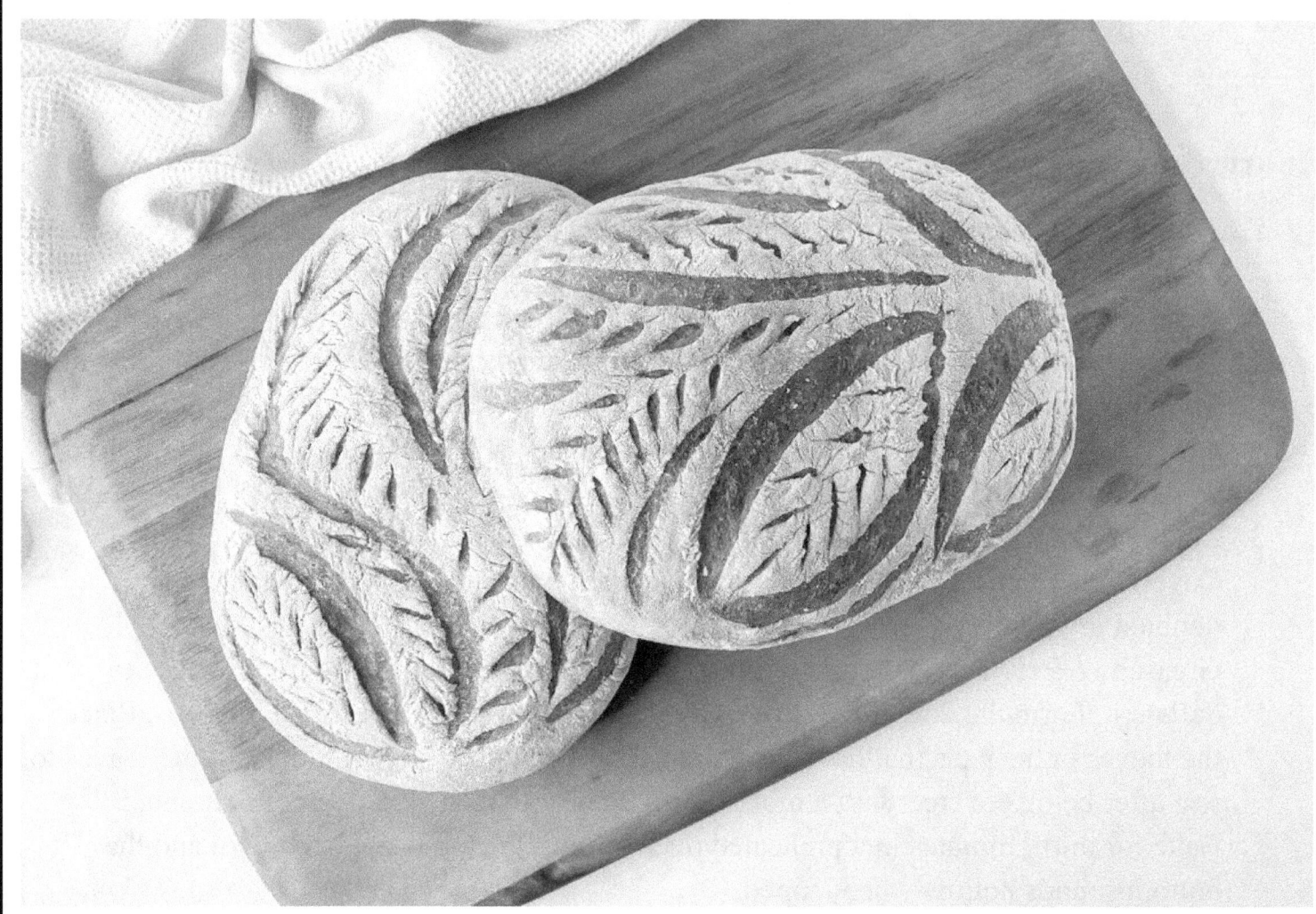

This is a really simple bread to make because it does not require any kneading. Bake in a sturdy casserole dish or a Dutch oven. The bread is really crusty and has many holes in it, just like at the bakery.

Nutrition

Calories: 230 | Protein: 6.7g | Fat: 0.7g | Sodium: 778.8mg | Carbohydrates 48g

Ingredients

- 1 teaspoon active dry yeast
- 1 teaspoon chopped fresh rosemary (Optional)
- 1 teaspoon chopped fresh sage (optional)
- 1 teaspoon chopped fresh thyme (optional)
- 1 ⅔ cups warm water
- 2 teaspoons salt
- 3 cups all-purpose flour

Instructions

1. In a large mixing dish, whisk together the flour, yeast, and salt. Mix in the water and, if using, the herbs. The dough will be quite sticky and shaggy in appearance. Cover the bowl with plastic wrap and set it aside for eighteen to twenty-four hours at room temperature.
2. Flour a work surface liberally. The dough will have risen and become bubble-covered. Dust the dough with flour and place it in the work area. Fold the dough in half and then roll it into a ball by stretching and tucking the dough's sides underneath it.
3. Flour a kitchen towel liberally. Place the floured towel on top of the dough ball. Cover with a floured towel once more. Allow for a two-hour rise time
4. Preheat the oven to 450 degrees Fahrenheit. Preheat the oven with a covered Dutch oven or a big heavy-duty casserole dish (with a lid).
5. Remove the hot baking dish from the oven with care. Remove the lid and carefully place the dough ball, seam-side up, in an ungreased baking dish; shake the dish to distribute the dough evenly.
6. Bake for thirty minutes with the lid on. Remove the lid and bake for fifteen to twenty minutes, or until the crust is golden brown. Before slicing, remove the bread from the baking dish and cool on a rack.

AUTHENTIC GERMAN BREAD (BAUERNBROT)

Preparation: 3 Hours

Cook: 2 Hours

Servings: 20

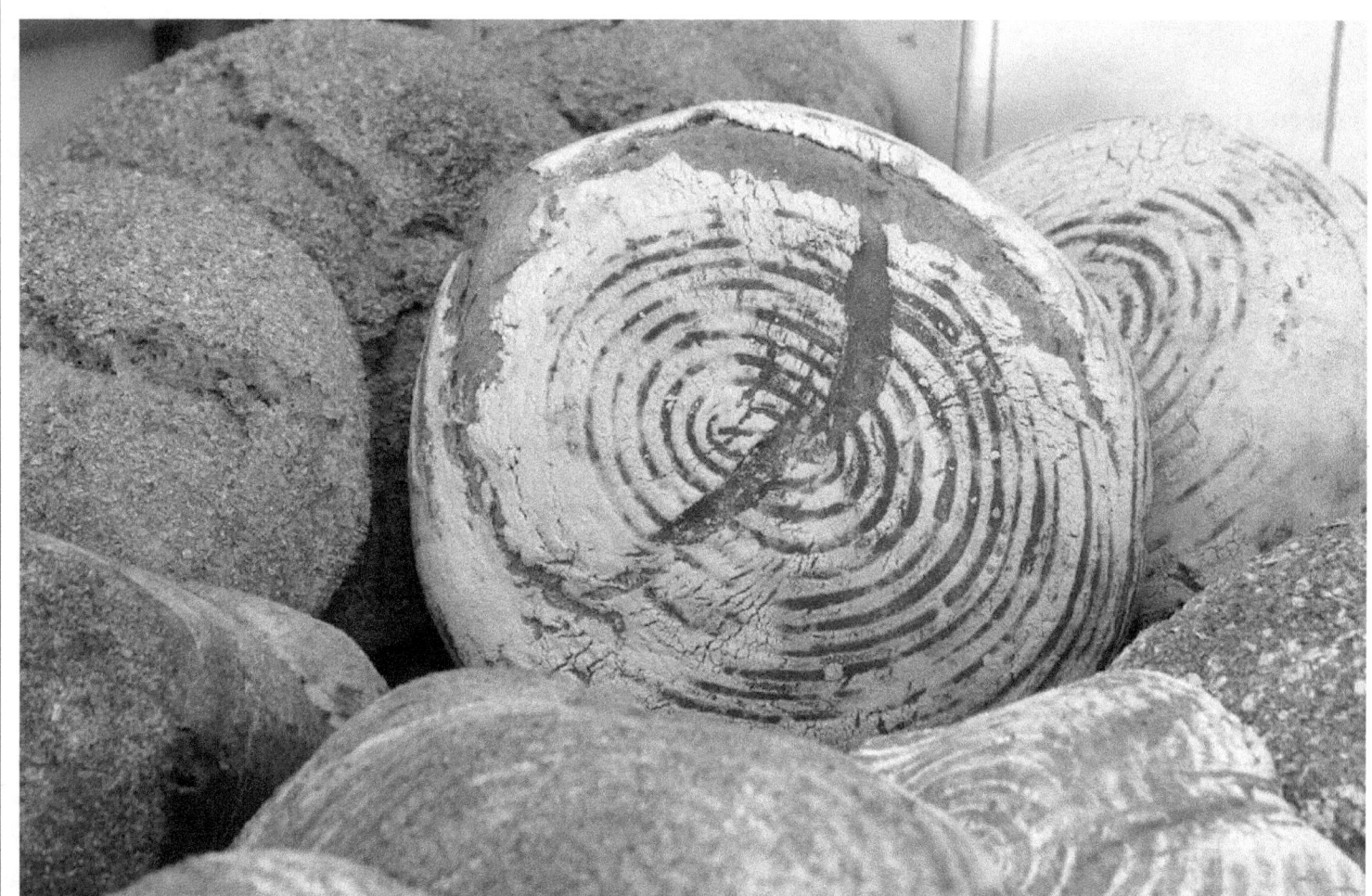

This is a fantastic recipe for traditional German sourdough bread. This bread tastes nearly identical to the bread we buy in Bavaria, Germany. They still make their bread once every two weeks in a very old stone oven in the center of a little community.

Nutrition

Calories: 334 | Protein: 9.2g | Fat: 1.3g | Sodium: 701.9mg | Carbohydrates: 71.6g

Ingredients

- 1-quart warm water
- 1 teaspoon white sugar
- 1 ½ ounce compressed fresh yeast
- 2 cups warm water
- 2 tablespoons salt
- 2 tablespoons white sugar
- 8 cups all-purpose flour, divided
- 8 cups white rye flour

Instructions

1. Make the sourdough starter first. In a large mixing bowl, crumble the yeast. 1-quart warm water and 2 tablespoons sugar, whisked together until sugar is dissolved. The water temperature should be just above body temperature. Whisk in 4 cups flour in a slow, steady stream until all lumps are gone. Cover with a dish towel and set aside at room temperature for twenty-four hours.
2. Stir thoroughly after twenty-four hours, cover, and set aside for another twenty-four hours. It will be a thin, light-colored sourdough that may be used immediately.
3. Mix the rye flour, remaining 4 cups of all-purpose flour, salt, and sugar in a large mixing dish. Using a wooden spoon, whisk in the sourdough starter, then 2 cups of warm water. Put the dough in a heavy-duty stand mixer to mix for the first couple of minutes, but if it can't handle the heavy dough, use your hand to turn it out onto a floured board.
4. It's best to have a clean countertop. If the dough is too stiff, add a few teaspoons of water at a time to knead it. Fold the dough over, pull it apart, do whatever it takes to knead it well. To achieve a smooth dough, allow fifteen to twenty minutes for kneading. Place the dough in a large mixing bowl, cover, and rest for one to two hours, or until doubled.
5. Scrape the dough out of the bowl and onto a floured board once it has risen. Knead for five minutes at a time. This is necessary in order to activate gluten. Form into one or two long loaves. Place on baking sheets and let rise for one hour, or until a gentle poke with your finger leaves an indentation on the bread.
6. Preheat oven to 425 degrees Fahrenheit. Bake the bread for forty-five minutes if you're making two loaves, one and half hours if you're making one large loaf. If the crust is dark, don't be concerned. The bread, as well as the crust, will be wonderful. Allow it to cool completely before slicing.

HONEY BUNCH BREAD

Preparation: 30 Minutes

Cook: 40 Minutes

Servings: 36

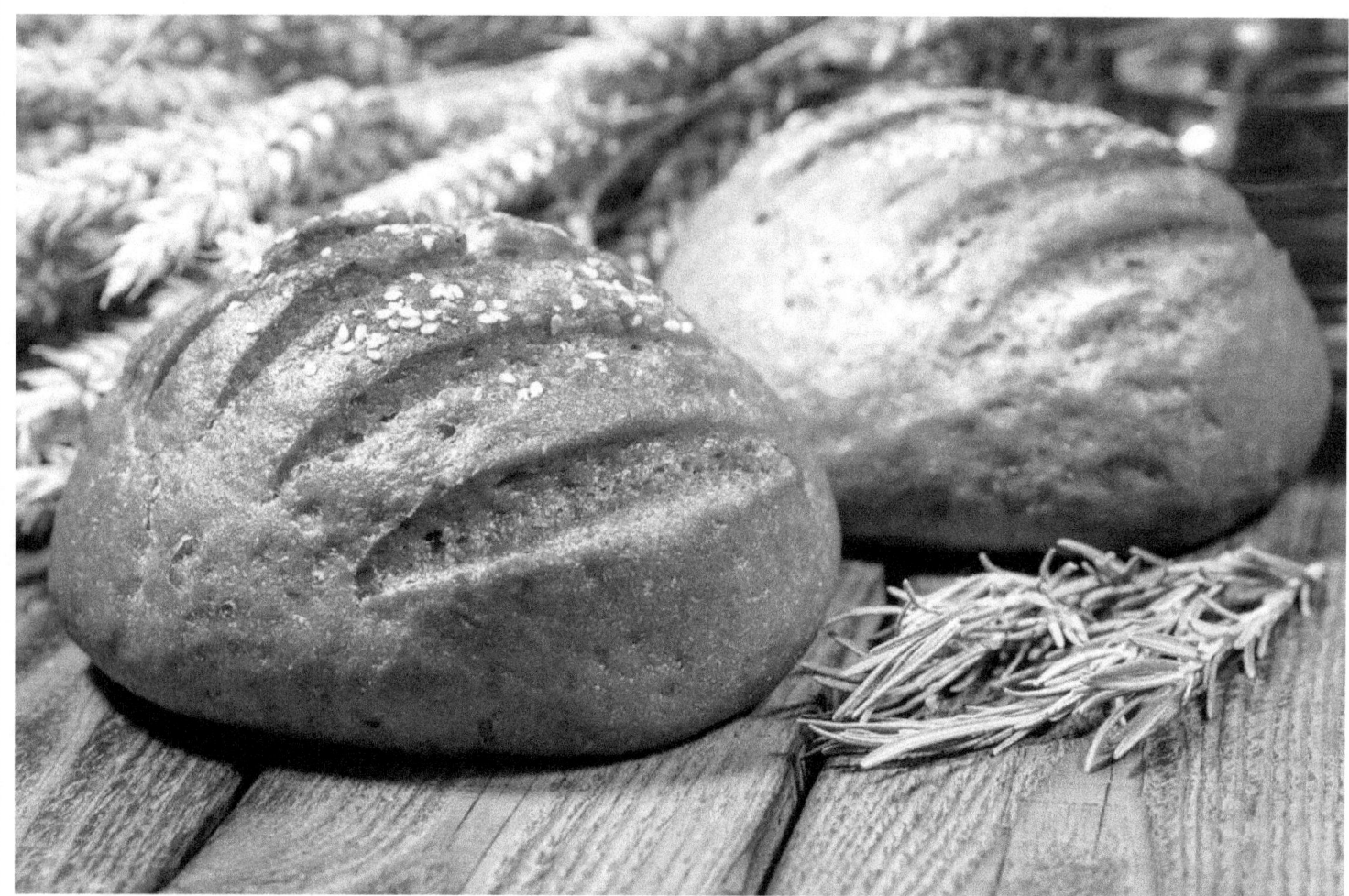

This is the best family favorite bread recipe, and it's even better with honey.

Nutrition

Calories: 110 | Protein: 2.4g | Fat: 2.3g | Sodium: 195.3mg | Carbohydrates 20g

Ingredients

- ⅓ cup vegetable oil
- ½ cup honey
- 1 tablespoon salt
- 2 tablespoons active dry yeast
- 2 ¾ cups warm water
- 6 cups all-purpose flour, or more as needed

Instructions

1. In a mixing dish, combine warm water and honey and stir until honey is completely dissolved. Allow five minutes for the yeast to soften and form a creamy foam after being sprinkled over the water mixture.
2. In a mixing bowl, combine the yeast, oil, and salt. 3 cups flour, sifted into the yeast mixture until there are no dry patches. Stir in the remaining flour, 1/2 cup at a time, until the dough is no longer sticky and pulls together, mixing well after each addition. Knead for another five minutes in a stand mixer or another ten minutes by hand.
3. Turn the dough into a big, lightly oiled dish to coat it. Cover bowl with a towel and set aside in a warm place to rise for one hour or until doubled in volume.
4. Allow dough to rise until it has doubled in bulk, about forty-five minutes.
5. Grease three 9x5-inch loaf pan
6. Punch down the dough and place it on a floured surface. Form the dough into three loaves and lay them in the pans that have been prepared. Cover loaves with a wet cloth and allow to rise for forty-five minutes, or until dough is about 1 inch above the sides of the loaf pans.
7. Preheat the oven to 350 degrees Fahrenheit.
8. Bake for forty minutes in a preheated oven until the tops are golden brown and the bottoms of the loaves sound hollow when tapped. Remove the loaves from the pans and place them on a cooling rack to cool.

CHEF JOHN'S CUBAN BREAD

Preparation: 25 Minutes

Cook: 20 Minutes

Servings: 12

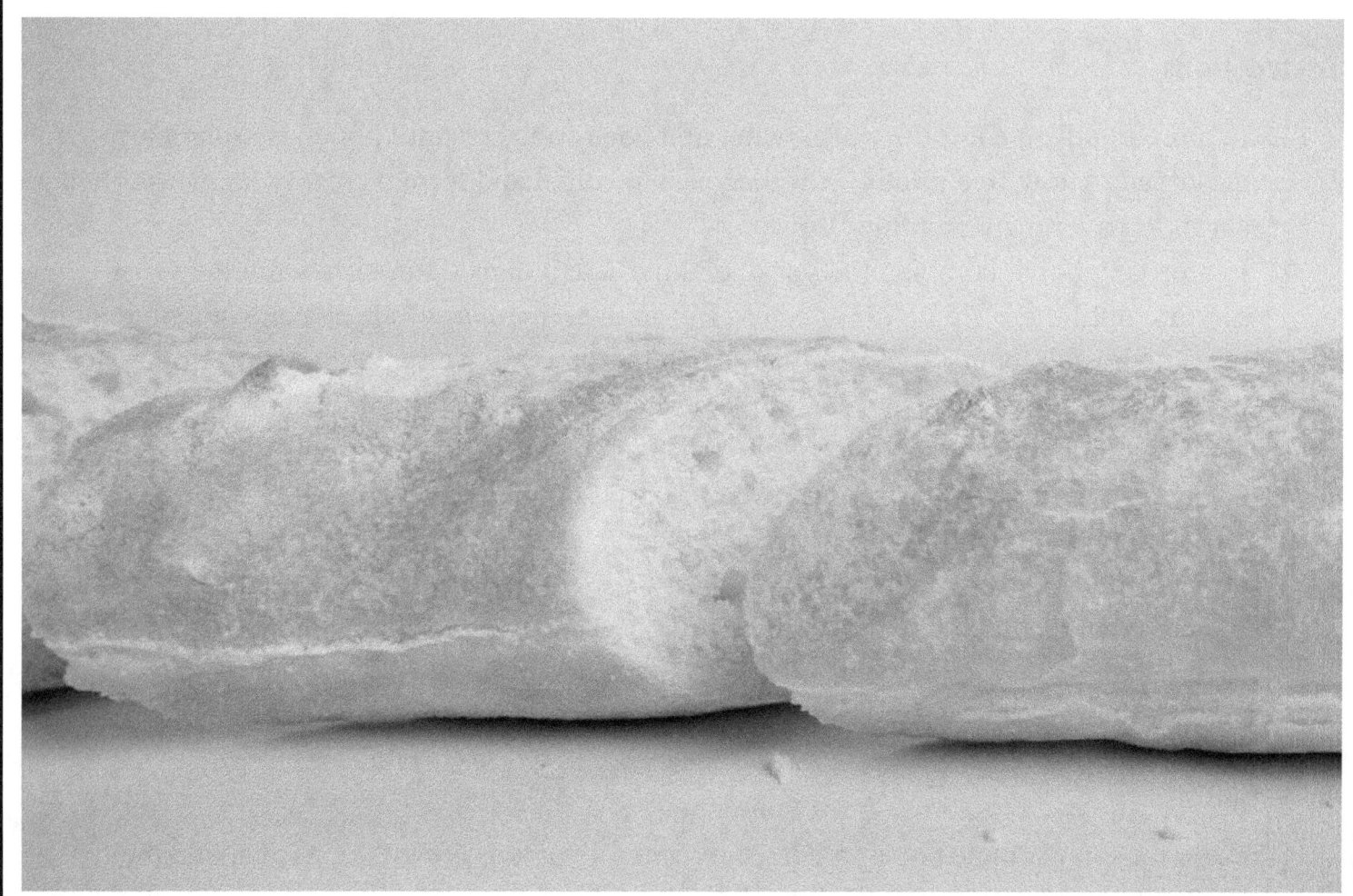

I didn't believe I loved Cuban sandwiches until I tried one made with authentic Cuban bread—wow! This bread is made with lard and a fermented starter, as well as a double dose of yeast. All of this contributes to the flavor and elevation of the dish.

Nutrition

Calories: 169 | Protein: 4.1g | Cholesterol: 3mg | Sodium: 389.5mg

Carbohydrates: 29.4g | Fat: 3.6g

Ingredients

Starter

- ½ cup flour
- ½ cup warm water
- ½ teaspoon active dry yeast

Dough

- ¾ cup warm water
- 1 package active dry yeast
- 1 tablespoon cornmeal
- 2 teaspoons fine salt
- 2 teaspoons white sugar
- 3 cups all-purpose flour, or as needed - divided
- 3 tablespoons lard
- Water to spray tops of loaves

Instructions

1. In a mixing bowl or measuring cup, combine 1/2 cup warm water, 1/2 teaspoon yeast, and 1/2 cup flour. Whisk the starter until it's completely combined. Refrigerate overnight, covered in plastic wrap.
2. In a mixing bowl, combine 1 package of active dry yeast and 2 teaspoons sugar. 3/4 cup warm water, poured in. Allow for a fifteen minutes rest period to confirm that the yeast is still alive. In a mixing bowl, combine the lard and salt; add 1 cup of the flour. Mix until all of the ingredients are combined, and the dough comes together into a sticky ball. If preferred, add the starter. Sprinkle the remaining flour on top of the dough, reserving 1/2 cup for kneading if necessary.
3. Knead the dough on a lightly floured work area until it comes together in a solid ball, only adding more flour as needed. The dough should be soft and elastic, with a slight tackiness on top.
4. Place the dough in a dish and lightly coat the surface with vegetable oil. Cover bowl with a moist dish towel and set aside to rise in a warm location. Allow rising for at least two hours, or until doubled in size.
5. Sprinkle a little cornmeal on two rimmed baking sheets lined with parchment paper.
6. Place dough on a floured work surface. With lightly greased hands, lightly press the dough into a rectangle. Divide the dough in half and flatten and shape each half into a 12-inch long 1/2-inch thick rectangle. To make a slim loaf, begin rolling from the long end.

7. Just a tiny little bit of flattening is required. Dust each loaf with flour and place it on a preheated baking sheet. Cover with a light, dry towel and let rise for one and half hours, or until doubled in size.
8. Preheat the oven to 400 degrees Fahrenheit. With a sharp knife or razor, cut a 1/4-inch deep incision over the top of the loaves. Lightly mist the loaves with water.
9. Place one pan on the lower rack and the other on the upper rack in a preheated oven. Switch pan positions after ten minutes. Bake for another ten to fifteen minutes, or until the loaves are golden brown. Place the loaves on a cooling rack to cool completely before slicing.

BLENDER WHITE BREAD

Preparation: 10 Minutes

Cook: 40 Minutes

Servings: 10

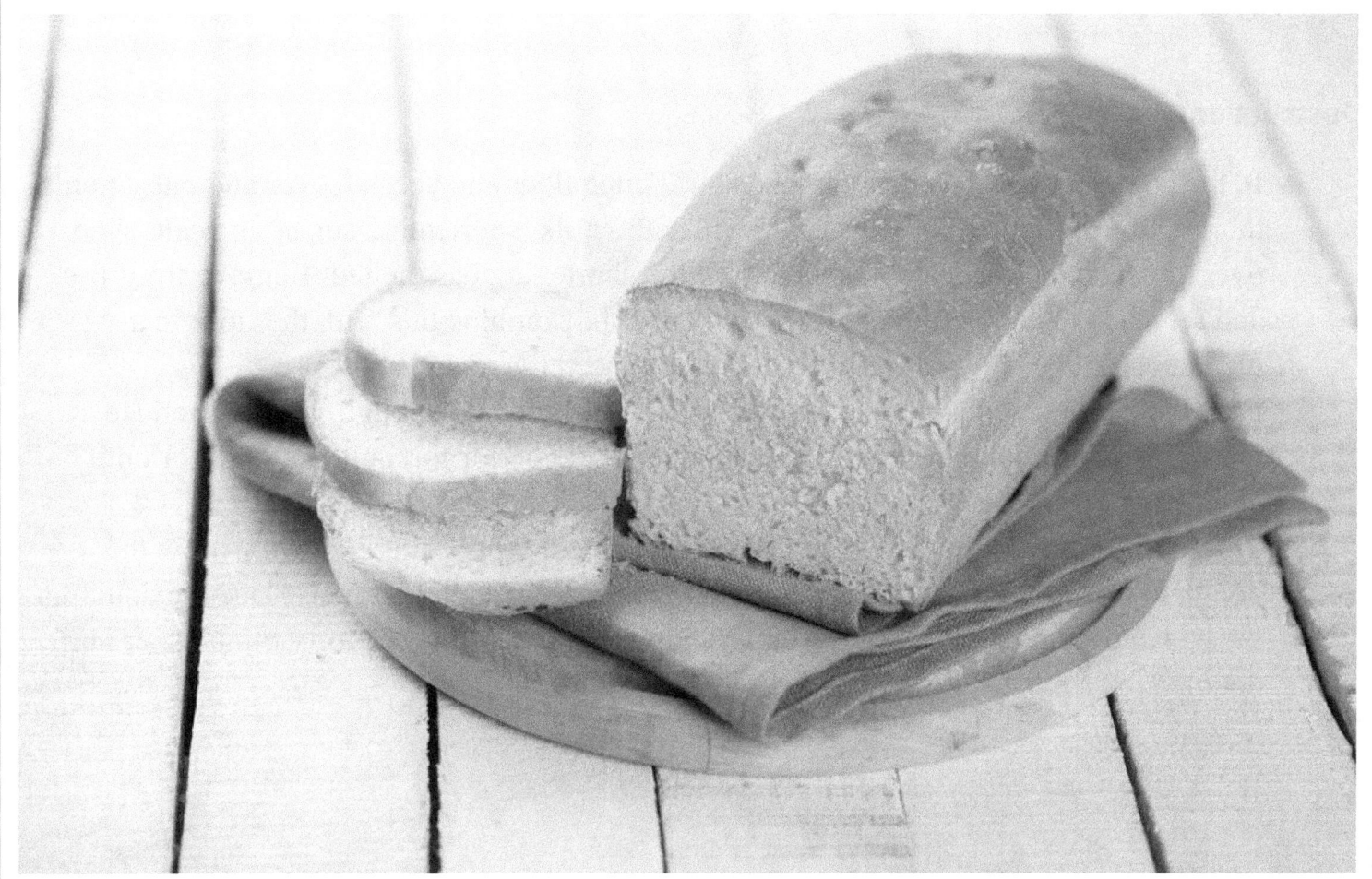

This is an easy-to-follow blender-style bread recipe that bakes up wonderfully.

Nutrition

Calories: 236 | Protein: 6.2g | Cholesterol: 20.6mg | Sodium 250.8mg

Carbohydrates: 37.3g | Fat: 6.6g

Ingredients

- ¼ cup shortening
- 1 package active dry yeast
- 1 cup milk
- 1 egg
- 1 teaspoon salt
- 2 tablespoons white sugar
- 3 ½ cups all-purpose flour, divided

Instructions

1. In the container of a blender, combine 1 1/2 cups flour and yeast. Cover and pulse until thoroughly combined. In a saucepan, whisk the milk, shortening, sugar, and salt. Warm over low heat, occasionally stirring, until the shortening has melted. Remove from fire and set aside to cool until just warm to the touch. Combine this with the flour in a blender. Add the egg and blend at the lowest speed to combine.
2. Pour the combined ingredients into a mixing bowl and add enough flour to produce a moderately firm dough. Cover with a cloth and let rise for forty-five minutes or until doubled in size.
3. Turn out the dough onto a lightly floured surface after punching it down. Allow the dough to rest for a few minutes while you grease a 9x5 inch loaf pan. Place the dough in the pan and shape it into a loaf. Allow rising for another thirty to forty minutes, or until doubled in size.

BUTTERMILK BREAD

Preparation: 20 Minutes

Cook: 35 Minutes

Servings: 24

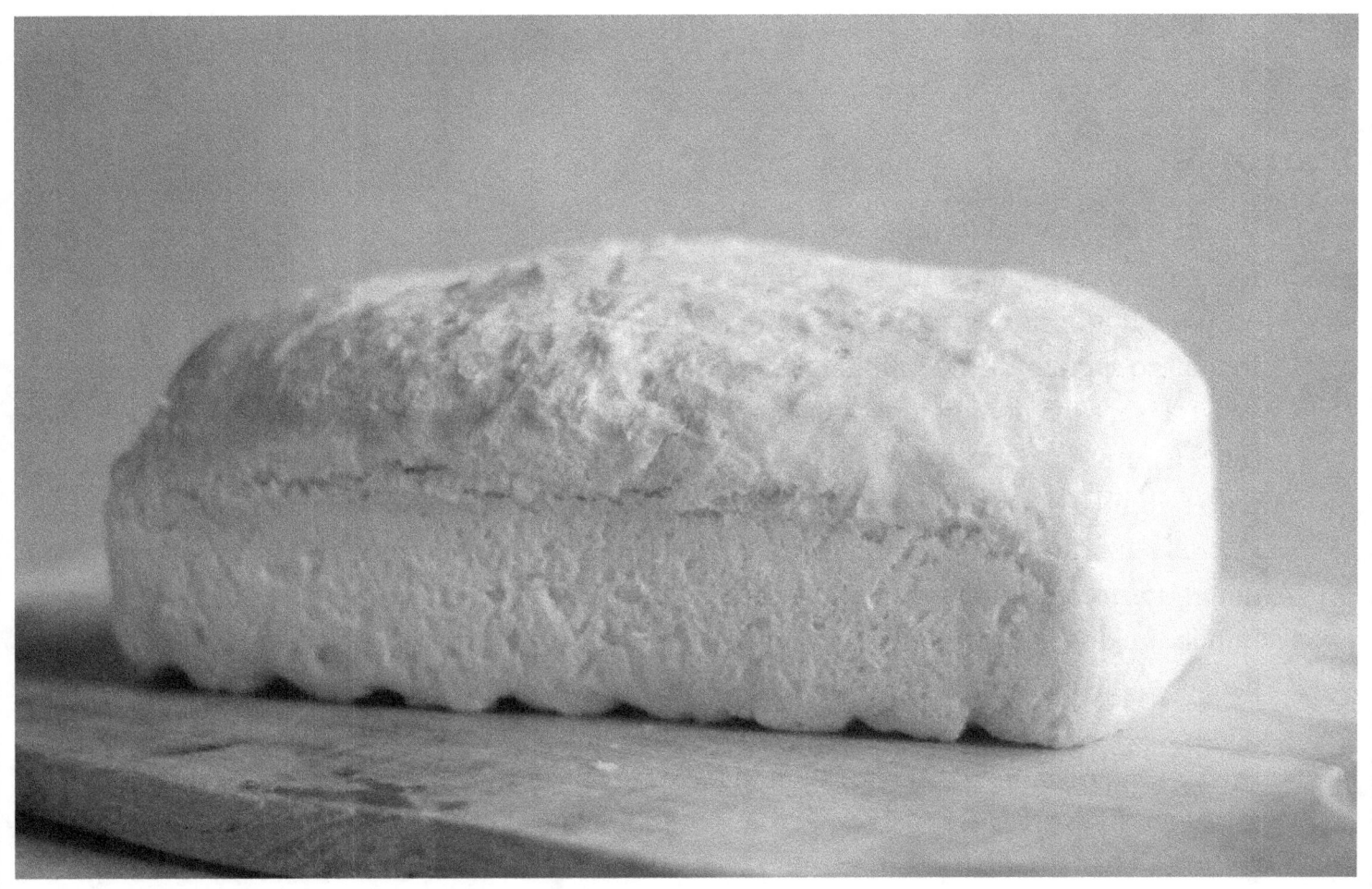

This bread tastes great, either plain or toasted. It really should be made at least once a week.

Nutrition

Calories: 49 | Protein: 0.8g | Cholesterol: 0.6mg | Sodium: 280.3mg

Carbohydrates: 3.1g | Fat: 3.9g

Ingredients

- ¼ cup white sugar
- ½ cup margarine
- ½ cup warm water
- ½ teaspoon baking soda
- 1 ½ cups buttermilk
- 2 packages of active dry yeast
- 2 teaspoons salt
- 5 ½ cups bread flour

Instructions

1. Warm water is used to proof yeast.
2. In a small saucepan, combine the butter or margarine and the buttermilk. Slowly heat until the butter or margarine has completely melted. Allow it to cool to lukewarm.
3. In a large mixing dish, combine the sugar, salt, baking soda, buttermilk mixture, and yeast. Using the dough hook attachment of an electric mixer, add 3 cups of flour one at a time. Continue to mix while gradually adding the remaining flour. Turn out the dough onto a lightly floured surface until it is no longer sticky. Knead the dough for several minutes or until it is soft and smooth. Turn once in a greased mixing bowl. Allow the dough to rise until it has doubled in size.
4. Punch the dough down. Divide the dough into two loaves. Place in two 8 x 4-inch bread pans that have been properly oiled. Allow dough to rise until it is one inch higher than the pans.
5. Preheat the oven to 375 degrees F and bake for thirty to thirty-five minutes. When knocked, the loaves should be pleasantly golden and hollow sounding.

TRADITIONAL WHITE BREAD

Preparation: 25 Minutes

Cook: 25 Minutes

Servings: 20

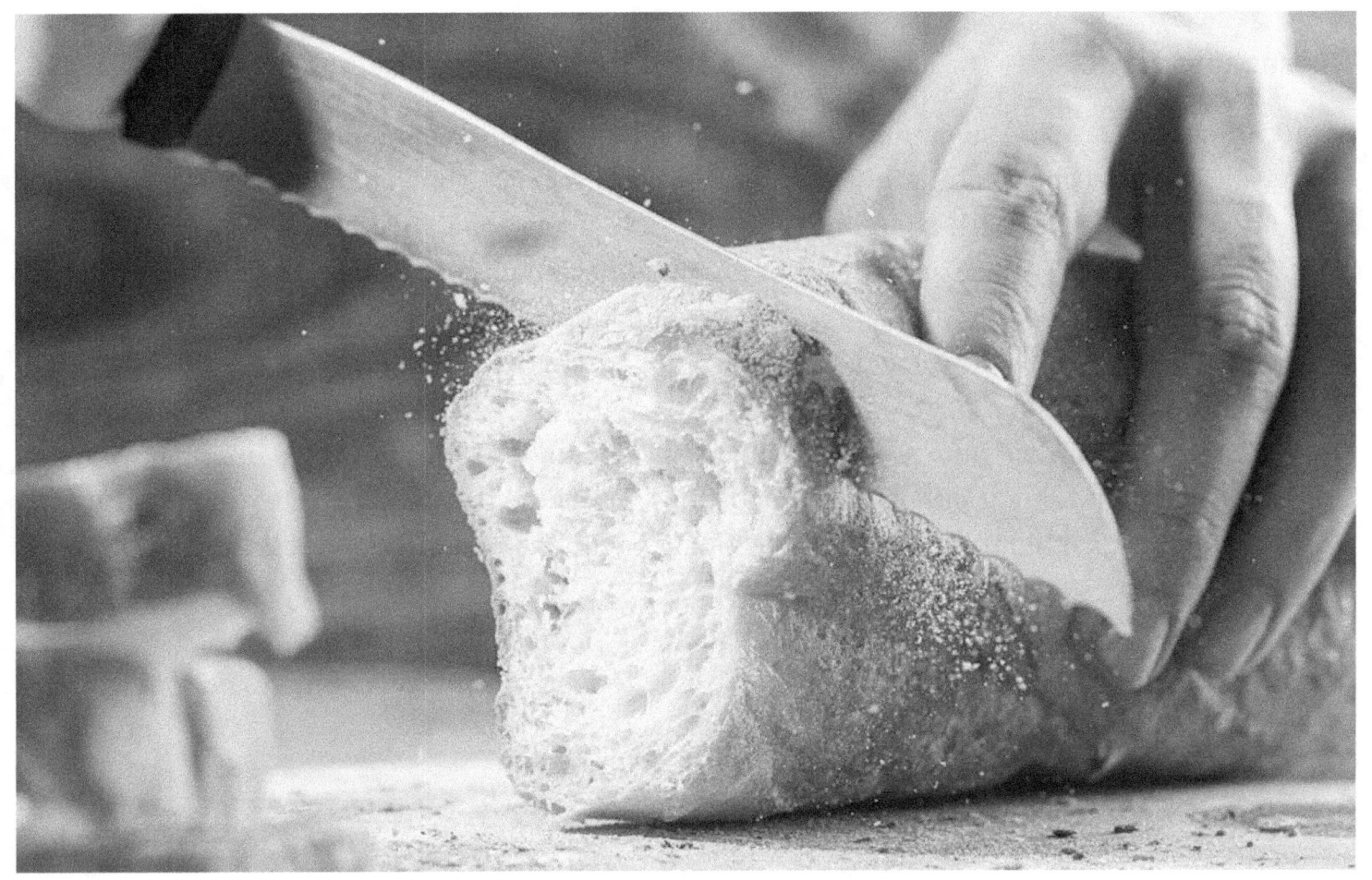

Great bread with a delicate, crunchy crust and a light inside. If you don't want to use lard, you can use butter or vegetable oil instead.

Nutrition

Calories: 167 | Protein: 4.8g | Cholesterol: 0.8mg | Sodium: 306.4mg

Carbohydrates: 26.2g | Fat: 1.7g

Ingredients

- 1 tablespoon salt
- 2packages active dry yeast
- 2 ½ cups warm water
- 3 tablespoons lard, softened
- 3 tablespoons white sugar
- 6 ½ cups bread flour

Instructions

1. Dissolve yeast and sugar in warm water in a large mixing container. Combine the lard, salt, and two cups of flour in a mixing bowl. 1/2 cup at a time, add the remaining flour, beating well after each addition. When the dough has come together, turn it out onto a lightly floured surface and knead for about eight minutes, or until smooth and elastic.
2. Lightly grease a large mixing bowl, then set the dough in it and turn to coat it in oil. Cover with a moist towel and set aside in a warm place to rise for one hour or until doubled in volume.
3. Turn the dough out onto a lightly floured surface to deflate it. Form the dough into two loaves by dividing it into two equal portions. Place the loaves in two 9x5-inch loaf pans that have been lightly oiled. Cover the loaves with a moist cloth and let rise for about forty minutes, or until doubled in volume.
4. Preheat the oven to 425 degrees Fahrenheit
5. Bake for thirty minutes at 375°F, or until the top is golden brown and the bottom of the loaf sounds hollow when tapped.

CIABATTA

Preparation: 20 Minutes

Cook: 20 Minutes

Servings: 15

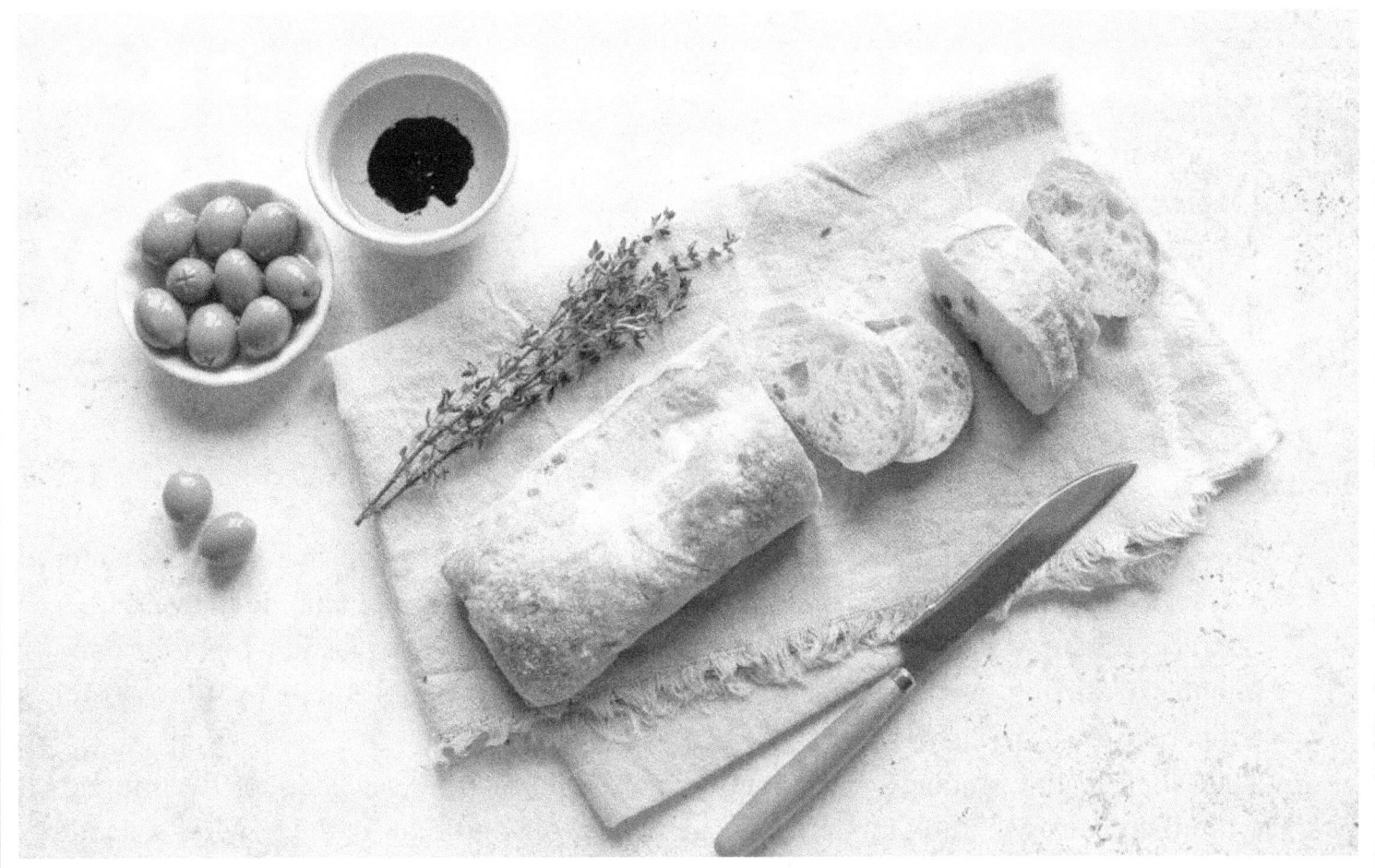

Make the starter, also known as sponge, in five minutes tonight, then bake two loaves of this wonderful, slightly sour, rustic Italian bread with a hearty crust tomorrow.

Nutrition

Calories: 96 | Protein: 3g | Cholesterol: 0.2mg | Sodium: 234.5mg

Carbohydrates: 17.6g | Fat: 1.3g

Ingredients

For Sponge (Biga)

- ⅛ teaspoon active dry yeast
- ⅓ cup warm water
- 1 cup bread flour
- 2 tablespoons warm water

For Bread

- ½ teaspoon active dry yeast
- ⅔ cup warm water
- 1 tablespoon olive oil
- 1 ½ teaspoons salt
- 2 cups bread flour
- 2 tablespoons warm milk

Instructions

1. To make the sponge: combine 1/8 teaspoon yeast with warm water in a small container and set aside for five minutes, or until creamy. In a mixing dish, combine the yeast mixture, 1/3 cup water, and 1 cup bread flour. Cover bowl with plastic wrap after four minutes of stirring. Allow sponge to sit for at least twelve hours and up to 1 day at room temperature.
2. To Make Bread: Combine yeast and milk in a small bowl and set aside for five minutes, or until creamy. Mix milk mixture, sponge, water, oil, and flour in the bowl of a standing electric mixer fitted with the dough hook on low speed until flour is just moistened; add salt and mix until smooth and elastic, about eight minutes. Cover dough with plastic wrap after scraping it into an oiled bowl.
3. Allow dough to rise at room temperature for one and half hours or until it has doubled in size. Cut the dough in half on a lightly floured work surface. Form each part into an uneven oval about 9 inches long on a parchment sheet. Dust tops with flour and dimple loaves with floured fingers. Using a wet kitchen towel, cover the loaves. Allow loaves to rise at room temperature for one and a half to two hours, or until about doubled in size.
4. Preheat the oven to 425 F and place a baking stone on the lowest oven rack at least forty-five minutes before baking the ciabatta.

5. Place 1 loaf on a rimless baking sheet, putting the long side of the loaf parallel to the baking sheets far edge. Line up the far edge of the baking sheet with the far edge of stone or tiles, and tilt the baking sheet to slide loaf with parchment onto the back half of stone or tiles.
6. Repeat with the remaining loaf on the front half of the stone. Ciabatta loaves will be baked for twenty minutes or until pale golden. Place the loaves on a wire rack to cool.

ONION BREAD

Preparation:30 Minutes

Cook:40Minutes

Servings:12

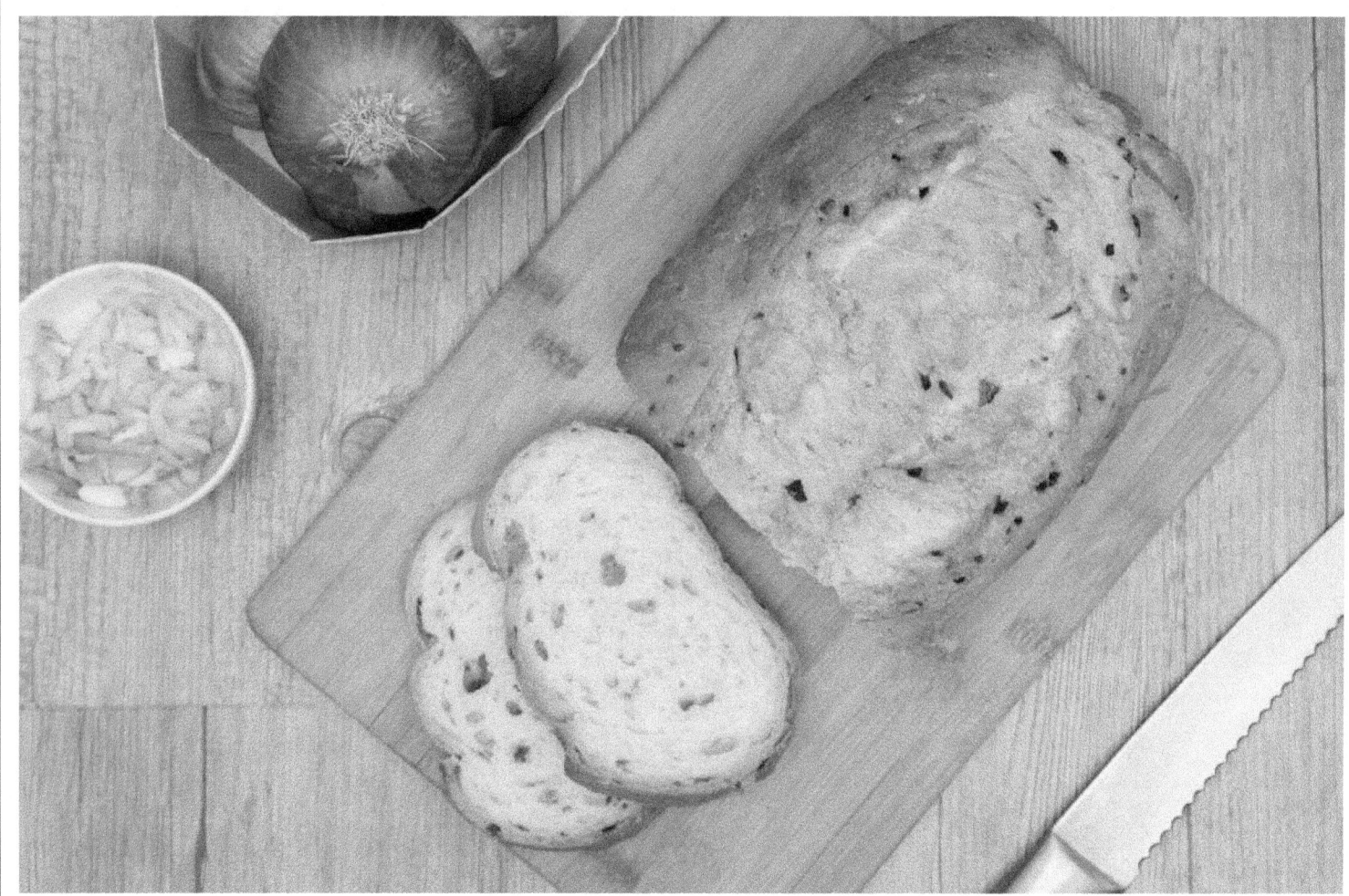

Onion bread from an old family recipe, baked to a golden brown and topped with onion circles. This is perfect for a ham sandwich.

Nutrition

Calories: 192 | Protein: 5.1g | Cholesterol: 5.1mg | Sodium: 402.5mg

Carbohydrates: 31.8g | Fat: 4.8g

Ingredients

- ½ onion
- ½ teaspoon dried oregano
- 1package active dry yeast
- 1 tablespoon minced onions
- 1 ½ cups warm water
- 2 tablespoons butter, melted
- 2 tablespoons shortening
- 2 tablespoons white sugar
- 2 teaspoons salt
- 3 ½ cups bread flour

Instructions

1. Dissolve yeast and sugar in warm water in a large mixing container. Allow ten minutes for the mixture to become creamy.
2. In a large bowl, whisk the yeast, shortening, minced onions, oregano, and 2 cups bread flour. 1/2 cup at a time, add the remaining flour, mixing well after each addition. Cover with a moist towel and set aside in a warm place to rise for one hour or until doubled in volume.
3. Deflate the dough and place it in a 9x5 inch loaf pan that has been lightly oiled. Cover with a wet cloth and let rise for about forty minutes, or until the top of the dough is within 1/2 inch of the pan's top. Preheat the oven to 375 degrees F in the meantime
4. Place onion slices on top of the bread after it has risen. Pour melted butter over the slices and bake for thirty-five to forty minutes, or until golden brown, in a preheated oven. Remove from the pan and set aside to cool on a wire rack.